Sexuality and Women
with Learning Disabilities

Michelle McCarthy

Foreword by Hilary Brown

Jessica Kingsley Publishers
London and Philadelphia

First published in the United Kingdom in 1999 by
Jessica Kingsley Publishers Ltd
116 Pentonville Road,
London N1 9JB,
England
and
325 Chestnut Street,
Philadelphia, PA 19106,
USA.

www.jkp.com

Copyright © 1999 Michelle McCarthy
Foreword Copyright © 1999 Hilary Brown

Library of Congress Cataloging-in-Publication Data
McCarthy, Michelle, 1962–
Sexuality and women with learning disabilities / Michelle McCarthy.
p.   cm.
Includes bibliographical references and index.
ISBN 1 85302 730 8 (pb : alk. paper)
1. Learning disabled women--United States--Sexual behavior.
2. Learning disabled women--Services for--United States. 3. Sexual harassment of women--United States. 4. Sex instruction for the learning disabled--United States. I. Title.
HQ30.5.M393   1999
306.7'087--dc21
98-45896

British Library Cataloguing in Publication Data
A CIP catalogue record for this book is available from the British Library

ISBN 1 85302 730 8

Printed and Bound in Great Britain by
Athenaeum Press, Gateshead, Tyne and Wear

Contents

Author's Acknowledgements

My thanks go to the many women and one man who have helped this book come to fruition. The women are: all those with learning disabilities with whom I have worked over many years, who have shared personal and often painful information with me; Helen Cosis Brown and Jeanne Gregory, who guided me so well through four years of doctoral research; Shona McEwan and the women artists from C.R.E.A.T.E., for the illustrations; Hilary Brown, for agreeing to write the foreword; and many other women colleagues who have indirectly supported my work through their own contributions to the field. The one man is David Thompson, who has always been generous with his help and support and whose work with men has both complemented and inspired mine with women.

Author's Note

The drawings which appear in Chapters Five and Six were done by women from C.R.E.A.T.E. (Creative Resources To Enable Artists To Enjoy): Jacqueline Blair, Carol Dickson, Rosemary Fawcett, Sheila McDonald and Wendy Muir. None of the women who drew pictures were involved in the research in any other way. C.R.E.A.T.E. can be contacted at the Woodlands Centre, Halbeath Road, Dunfermline, Scotland KY11 5EU.

Foreword

It is a privilege to be asked to write a foreword to this book. It offers a powerful account of the lives of women with learning disabilities and of their struggles to lead sexual lives which meet their needs. As the author says, the body of work dealing with sexuality and people with learning disabilities has often bypassed the views of women or men with learning disabilities themselves. For that reason, I had thought to begin by saying that the book was *over*due. But perhaps the reality is that it could not have been written until a number of barriers to listening and thinking had been cleared out of the way. Some of those barriers reflected ideological splits – fears that criticisms of life in the community might provoke an indiscriminate retreat into institutionalised service provision; reticence about naming abusive relationships as sexual abuse; a naïve commitment to choice at all costs without an analysis of power and powerlessness. All these have created white noise which has prevented the voices of individual women and men from being heard. And while it is possible that all these barriers were placed in the way with the best of intentions, there is no doubt that the time has come to look clearly at the way these issues are lived, rather than theorised about, and to place the voices of women with learning disabilities centre stage.

Michelle McCarthy's work provides a model in terms of research methodology and deserves to be read from that angle as well as for its content. Her interviews with the women are respectful and predicated on the need to 'give something back'. Her study is one of a growing number of studies using qualitative methodologies such as case studies, biographical and life history approaches, and intensive interviewing to complement and challenge more traditional overviews. Of course, there are risks in generalising from such in-depth work and the author is appropriately cautious about ascribing universality to the accounts she presents here, but she supports her conclusions with sound knowledge gleaned from many years' experience of working with women and, particularly, women with learning disabilities. Where accurate information is not available, people act on the basis of hunches or projections. Whether their inclination is to shelter and protect or to champion individual rights and freedoms, they may do so either or both on the basis of unfounded assumptions. She finds, for example, that community-based services do not provide easy answers or improved opportunities and that the world for women with learning disabilities has 'both changed hugely and hardly at all'. The book poses some clear challenges to service providers, including the need to:

- recognise the disadvantages women with learning disabilities encounter in their sexual relationships with men and not hide behind cosy assumptions

- assure the rights to, visibility of, and respect for lesbian relationships

- provide safe placements and work to prevent sexual abuse

- re-evaluate the quality of social life and relationships in community settings

- re-state the commitment to maintaining personal space and privacy

- change the law and workings of the criminal justice system to ensure that women with learning disabilities have *at least* the same level of protection and redress as other women.

It also provides a challenge to activists in the disability and women's movements as to why both movements should have marginalised women with learning disabilities. The strength of the book lies in the author's insightful analysis and feminist commitment, and in its fluency and moral clarity. It is both scholarly and direct. It is often observed that one cannot see the wood for the trees, but when it comes to sex people often skirt around the wood *ad infinitum*. Here we see individual trees: real women's lives, and the compromises and contradictions they give rise to on the part of service providers – the wood will not look the same again. As Michelle McCarthy writes: 'What seems very clear is that few women would be satisfied with what is offered to most women with learning disabilities'. This book will help to inform all of those who bear the responsibility for changing that rather depressing reality.

Hilary Brown
Open University
November 1998

Introduction

'Women with learning disabilities are women too' (Williams 1992, p.149). This fact and its implications, now so obvious and important to me, has not always been at the forefront of my mind, even during the period when I was most active in feminist politics and organisations. From the mid- to late-1980s, I was either working full-time with people with learning disabilities or training to be a social worker with a view to returning to the learning disability field. During this time I was also closely involved with a small group of other women in setting up and running a rape crisis service in our town. I was also part of a support group for the local Women's Aid refuge. At that time I considered my work with women on issues of violence and sexual abuse, and my work with people with learning disabilities, to be two completely separate areas of interest. Nobody I knew, nor anything I read at that time, suggested otherwise. However, once I facilitated my first group for women with learning disabilities, my eyes were opened to the fact that, particularly with regards to sexual abuse, those women had much in common with other women.

From that point on, I began to see many connections (and some differences) and my working life changed. During my social work practice I became increasingly interested in supporting women with learning disabilities in their personal and sexual relationships and this led to me taking up a post which was solely concerned with issues related to sexuality and learning disabilities. By the time the research for this book began in 1992, I had been employed for three years as the team leader of a small specialist sex education team for people with learning disabilities. As the only woman on the team, I was responsible for all individual and group work with women with learning disabilities. My work covered a broad range of issues related to sexuality, such as: safer sex education; support and counselling regarding relationships and sex; sexual abuse prevention work; counselling and support for women who had been abused; and sex education in the commonly understood sense of the term.

My direct work experience on this team, and a small piece of academic research based on it (McCarthy 1991), had given me some good insights into how women with learning disabilities were experiencing their sexual lives. However, it was noticeable that the growing body of literature regarding sexuality and learning disability did not explore or describe the reality of actual sexual experiences of actual women and men. Rather, the literature was 'about sexuality' in a more abstract sense. In Chapters One and Two of this book I have set my own work in the context of the literature on sexuality and learning disability as well as in the context of research and thinking on sexuality issues more broadly.

My motivation for conducting the research, then, was to fill the gaps in my own knowledge but also to fill the gaps in 'knowledge' in a wider sense. My motivation for writing this book was to make my findings and analysis available to others working in the field in the hope that a greater understanding about the sexual lives of women with learning disabilities would lead to them being offered better support than they had hitherto received.

I was very aware at the outset of the research that it would probably not benefit the seventeen respondents themselves in any direct way. However, this is not unusual in research and it is not necessarily problematic or unethical as long as both the researcher and researched are clear about it:

> ... it should be noted that even if research has little impact on the lives of those included in it, it may be important for the category of persons they are taken to represent. Thus, work on rape, or women's housing problems may be too late to alleviate the suffering of those directly involved in it, but can contribute to legislation, policy or the behaviour of agencies in ways which later enhance the experiences of others. (Maynard 1994, p.17)

Although it is true that the women involved in this research will probably not profit in any way from the end results of it, nevertheless I was confident that they could benefit from the process. I was also anxious to avoid the situation of being overly intrusive with relative strangers (bearing in mind the nature of the investigation). I therefore made a commitment that I would not talk to any women with learning disabilities purely for research purposes. This meant that I arranged all seventeen interviews to take place in the context of my providing the women with educational or counselling support on relationship/sexuality issues. There is a full discussion in Chapter Three on methodology and methods.

Using semi-structured in-depth interviews, I have obtained information from seventeen women with learning disabilities on the following areas:

- the range of sexual activities they engage in
- their preferences and dislikes in relation to that
- their knowledge about their bodies
- decision making and control over sexual activity
- coerced or forced sexual activities
- their sex education
- their impressions of other people's sexual lives
- their sexual and reproductive health, including their use of contraception.

The main findings (presented in full in Chapter Four) are that only a small minority of the women were very positive about their sexual lives. The majority lacked control in terms of deciding for themselves what they wanted to do, with whom, when and how. Most of the women experienced exclusively or predominantly penetrative sex. A lack of sexual pleasure generally, and of orgasm specifically, was reported by all the women. In addition, very high levels of sexual abuse were reported. In Chapter Five the findings of this research are discussed in the context of other related work in the learning disability field and other research on the sexuality and sexual abuse of non-disabled women. One of the most important findings is that, with a few exceptions, there was relatively little difference in the experiences of women who lived, or had lived, in hospitals when compared to women who lived in community settings. The quality of the women's experiences was more directly determined by the nature of the relationships they had with men, whether men were abusive or aggressive towards them, the women's level of self-esteem and assertiveness, and the availability of sex education and support.

The political context of this research is one whereby I have tried to make explicit how women with learning disabilities have, by and large, been rendered invisible in two human rights struggles, where they have a rightful place – namely the women's movement and the movement towards normalisation/social progress for people with learning disabilities. In this research study I have sought to rectify these omissions. In Chapter One I argue that it is due to feminist activism, research and scholarship that it is possible to recognise and challenge the sexual oppression of women. However, I also argue that much feminist analysis and many feminists have traditionally ignored the very existence of women with learning disabilities.

It has fallen to those of us who work within the learning disability field, and who are also feminists, to make 'mainstream' feminists aware of the experiences of women with learning disabilities. Encouraging and facilitating women with learning disabilities to speak out for themselves has been an important part of this process. In Chapter Two I argue that although the principles of normalisation and ordinary living have been of enormous importance in services for people with learning disabilities, they have, like the less helpful ideologies which preceded them, tended to obscure gender inequalities (and, indeed, inequalities based on race, sexual orientation and class) (Brown and Smith 1989,1992). Sexual rights have rightly had a fairly prominent place in the general demand for rights for people with learning disabilities. My work (and that of others) has demonstrated the necessity of recognising the gendered sexual lives that people tend to live and has spelt out what the implications of this are for many women with learning disabilities. These are highlighted in Chapters Four, Five and Six.

One of the important theoretical contributions of this work, then, is that I have used a methodology which makes analyses along the axes of both gender and disability. This is important because it has been argued that:

> ...the intersection of feminism and disability studies has been one of the least explored because of the dominance of disability as the primary category of analysis and the avoidance of feminist studies to include disability in their categories of difference. This process, whereby women with disabilities have fallen through the gaps of definition, theory, and consciousness, has manufactured a silence around them and their experiences. (Chenoweth 1996, p.394)

I wanted to avoid an analysis of the experiences of women with learning disabilities which suggested that any oppression stemmed purely from their gender. I also wanted to avoid some of the familiar traps of some research from a disability rights perspective: accepting a male norm and marginalising the concerns of disabled women (Morris 1996); and being firmly rooted in, and relating exclusively or primarily to, the experience of people with physical disabilities (see Chapter Three for further discussion).

The research reported in this book has taken place during a time of considerable change in services for people with learning disabilities and in the wider context. But the change process has been far from smooth. The large institutions for people with learning disabilities have continued to close but community-based provision continues to be under-resourced. In addition, there has been the introduction of the 'internal market' in the NHS and the development of NHS Trusts. Care Management and assessment have also been introduced in the social care market, which has become increasingly fragmented (Cambridge and Brown 1997; Wistow *et al.* 1994). Far more research is needed to monitor the effects of the various social policy changes upon the lives of individuals with learning disabilities (Stenfert Kroese, Gillot and Atkinson 1998). There is a widespread assumption that all aspects of life are fundamentally different depending on whether a person lives in a large institution or small community-based setting, with the community being always assumed as superior to the institution. A comparison between institutional and community settings has been an explicit feature of the research for this book and my findings suggest that with regards to one aspect of life, namely sexual experiences of women with learning disabilities, there are far fewer differences than might have been expected. Despite this, I am very clear in my discussion (Chapter Five) and recommendations (Chapter Six) why this particular finding should not be used in any way to argue for the continued provision of hospital-based services.

Working from a feminist perspective (integral to which is a belief that many sexual problems are a result of socially constructed gender roles and expectations), I anticipated that any recommendations resulting from this research would be in the realm of the social or political rather than the individual or private sphere. Indeed, this is what has transpired – whilst some of the recommendations in Chapter Six suggest changes that individual women with learning disabilities might be enabled to make, most of the recommendations involve steps to dismantle the wider, structural forms of oppression that the women face. The necessity for focusing on the social, and not the individual, context is demonstrated by taking a historical perspective. Whilst it is true that attitudes towards the sexuality of people with learning disabilities have improved over time, in the sense that they are not as punitive as they once were (Chapter Two), at another level it is also true to say that little has changed. The vulnerability of women with learning disabilities to sexual assault remains the same – take this quote from over a century ago: 'The feeble-minded woman...becomes the easy prey of man's lust' (Brown 1887, cited in Trent 1994, p.76). Writers today, myself included, are saying essentially the same thing, only using more up-to-date language. Of course, what has changed is that the solutions to the problem suggested today are different to those of a century ago. Brown's answer to the problem in 1887 was to lock up and/or supervise the women so they could not be sexually assaulted, whereas most people today would suggest locking up and/or supervising the perpetrators. However, that is not to say that the victims of sexual assault are never blamed or punished in learning disability services *any more* – that would be far from the truth (see McCarthy 1998b for a recent example).

Trent (1994) also describes how at dances in learning disability institutions at the turn of the century, male residents would have to dance with selected female staff whilst female residents would have to dance with each other. The assumption that any such contact between men with learning disabilities would automatically be sexual, and, therefore, inappropriate, has certainly not disappeared (see Thompson 1994b, p.259, for a modern, but nevertheless shocking, example of discrimination against two men with learning disabilities who wanted to dance together). The other assumptions operating in the Trent example are that women with learning disabilities would not be sexually interested in each other, which is still a prevalent notion (see Chapter Five for discussion of lesbian sexuality), and also that it was appropriate for women staff to act as surrogate partners for men with learning disabilities. The ambiguities and complexities surrounding the role of women staff in relation to the sexuality of men with learning disabilities are still far from resolved today (Thompson, Clare and Brown 1997).

The intention of this book is, therefore, to give some insight into the sexual lives of women with learning disabilities in a world which has both changed hugely and hardly at all.

CHAPTER ONE

Perspectives on Sexuality
and Sexual Violence

In order to put ideas about the sexuality and sexual abuse of women with learning disabilities into a broader context, it is necessary briefly to review current and historical thinking on the subjects of sexuality and learning disability, both separately and together. This chapter, therefore, looks first at a broad view of sexuality before moving on to a more specifically feminist perspective on sexuality issues.

Perspectives on sexuality

The traditional Western religious perspective on sexuality was that it is based on an impulse of the flesh, which resulted in, and from, humanity's fall from grace. The sexual impulse was seen as essentially evil in its nature and so powerful that it had to be kept under strict control. As Petras (1973) explains, this Western Judeo-Christian tradition inevitably set up a dichotomy between body and mind, with the body the site of physical desire and corruption and the mind the centre of spirituality and purity. Although religion has gradually lost its authority within many Western societies, some important features of this tradition can be seen in other perspectives.

One of the most influential perspectives on sexuality in the twentieth century has been the psychoanalytical perspective. Freud's model shares many features with traditional Christianity: sexuality is seen as a powerful instinct, opposed by its very nature to civilisation. Society, through social relationships and restraints, must work to psychologically repress the individual's instincts. As Freud himself put it 'civilization is built upon the renunciation of instinct' (1979, p.34). However, complete repression of the sexual instinct was not the only mechanism and diverting or channelling instincts into harmless or otherwise productive pursuits was also thought necessary within this framework.

Another perspective, that of the people who were sometimes labelled 'sexual radicals', like Wilhelm Reich, also looked at the interface between sexuality and society but came to quite different conclusions. Their model, sometimes called the 'therapeutic truth' model, also believed that sexuality was a powerful instinct but maintained that it was a fundamentally good and healthy instinct. Rather than society or civilisation being threatened by sexuality, as in the Freudian and Christian models, this model sees society as the negative force which distorts and represses a 'naturally' good human impulse (Reich 1969). This model has its roots in the Enlightenment era of the eighteenth century, where influential thinkers of the time argued 'that nature was good and that proper behaviour should seek to realise human nature rather than to dent, fight and conquer it' (Porter 1982, p.4).

Another variation on the theme of sexuality as a strong instinct is that propounded by Szasz (1980). Once again the case is made for sexuality as a powerful biological drive – next to the needs for water, food and sleep, *the* most powerful of human instincts. However, unlike the other perspectives, Szasz believes that neither releasing nor inhibiting the sexual drive causes any great harm.

A quite different, and, in fact, totally opposing perspective, is the social construction, or cultural learning, model proposed by, amongst others, Gagnon (1977) and Gagnon and Simon (1974). This is based on the premise that there is no sex drive or instinct but that people learn to be sexual in the same way that they learn to be and do everything else (or, put another way, if we want to think in terms of a sex drive, it does not drive us, we drive it). This process of learning to be sexual happens through what Gagnon and Simon call 'scripts'. Scripts involve both external, interpersonal factors such as mutually shared conventions and internal, intrapsychic factors such as motivation or arousal. Seen from this perspective, sex is no different from any other kind of behaviour and sexual feelings no more powerful and uncontrollable than any other kind of feelings. Gagnon (1977) argues that the special status given to sex in society is a self-fulfilling prophesy – that is, people experience sex as special because they have been taught to believe that it *is* special.

More than any of the other perspectives on sexuality, this one, which refers to the social construction of sexuality, has, in my view, the most validity and, of course, I am not alone in this conclusion (Foucault 1990; Plummer 1982; Jackson 1978). Weeks (1986) also makes a strong challenge to sex being 'an irresistible natural energy' with his argument that 'sexuality only exists through its social forms and social organisation' (p.24).

In my opinion, the social construction view makes most sense intellectually and offers a 'more compelling case' for a 'rich understanding' of human sexuality (Tiefer 1995, p.29). Specifically in the context of my research on the sexuality of women with learning disabilities, the concept of scripts seems to explain why so many women with learning disabilities describe their sexual activity as physical/mechanical/matter-of-fact encounters, rather than with any suggestion of the erotic/sexual. Gagnon suggests that for a sexual response, a person has to actively give sexual meanings to the event/stimuli in question. People have to go through a process of learning that certain things in certain contexts are meant to be sexual before they become sexual. It is my contention that, perhaps, many women with learning disabilities either have not learned sexual scripts and /or vital elements of the scripts (e.g. privacy, ability to fantasise or transfer knowledge or feelings from one situation to another) may be missing. There is a full discussion of this in Chapter Five.

The social construction perspective on sexuality maintains that sex is no more important than any other kind of behaviour, pointing out, moreover, that sexual activity itself occupies very little of most people's time and energy. Apart, perhaps, from those who work full time in the sex industry, most people spend most of their time not having sex. However, in modern Western societies sex itself, as well as sexual attractiveness and sexual feelings, are marketable commodities. Consequently, sex and sexuality are very visible features in society and, therefore, assume an importance greater than would otherwise be the case. Within the context of my work with women with learning disabilities, these ideas also make sense – they are amongst those people who tend to have less access to, and who, perhaps, make less sense of, overt sexual imagery. Also, along with the elderly or people with physical disabilities, they are usually not considered to be, nor are they publicly portrayed as, sexually attractive. It should not come as a surprise, therefore, to find that – based on their own reports and on my observations and understanding – sex is *not* an important part of the lives of most of the women with learning disabilities I have talked to (see p.201).

Sexology

At its simplest, sexology can be defined as the study of human sexual behaviour. But, as most things relating to sex are complex and controversial, we would not expect the study of sex to be as straightforward as the above definition implies. Claims have been made that sexology is 'impartial, empirical and in the manner of all sciences, non-judgemental' (Money 1988, p.6). However, there is, in fact, often little or no distinction between merely studying and reporting how people have sex and advocating how they should have sex: 'Sexology, then is not simply descriptive. It is at times profoundly prescriptive, telling us what we ought to be like, what makes us truly ourselves and "normal"' (Weeks 1991, p.74).

One of the ways sexology has successfully managed to be prescriptive, whilst presenting itself as scientific and objective, is because as a discipline it assumed a legitimacy through its associations with accepted institutions of power – for example, the law, but, more often, medicine. Foucault (1990) has described how power can be exercised through an interest in sexuality: defining and classifying categories of sexual interest can lead to turning the sexual behaviours and the people who carry them out into subjects for control. This is because these classifications do not go into a vacuum but, rather, are absorbed by people and institutions who already hold opinions and prejudices. Sexology, or, rather, the findings of sexologists, can be used by others for political purposes – that is, the development of new social or legal sanctions against those behaviours and people who are seen to be deviant. The clearest example of this, which Weeks (1985, 1989b) has written extensively about, is the development of the category 'homosexual'. Prior to the second half of the nineteenth century, having sex with a person of the same sex did not have any great significance to the way the person viewed themselves or others. It did not make you a particular kind of person and the word 'homosexual' was not invented until 1869 (by the Hungarian Benkert von Kertbeny). However, with the growing scientific interest at that time in differentiating and classifying things, it was only a matter of time before the 'homosexual' came to be seen as a distinct kind of person. Foucault (1990) described the process in the following way: 'The sodomite had been a temporary aberration; the homosexual was now a species' (p.43).

Influential sexologists

Although there had always been religious treatises on sexual matters throughout history, it was not until the eighteenth century that secular writings on sexuality started to appear, with Tissot's *On Onania* (a 1758 essay warning of the dangers of masturbation) probably the most well-known example. However, it was not until the last decades of the nineteenth and the beginning of the twentieth century that the discipline of sexology really developed. Ellis is generally credited as being *the* major influential thinker and writer at this time. His work emphasised the importance of researching the sexual lives of ordinary people and not just those of sexual offenders, people in mental asylums or therapy, as previous work in the field had done. He sought to measure normal sexual behaviour because he believed (quite rightly) that you could not say what was abnormal – statistically or otherwise – until you knew what was normal. His considered view on homosexuality, for example, was that it was a congenital condition and abnormal only in the sense of being statistically rare. Ellis' work was rooted in, and reflected, the social and political movements of his time. He was a strong supporter of eugenics and supported women's rights to equality, but only within certain limits. Although he has been credited as inventing a new kind of feminism, his work has been strongly criticised by feminists – a point I shall return to later.

Ellis died in 1939, just as Kinsey was beginning his sexological research, which was to become enormously influential, especially in the USA. His method of research was to conduct large-scale statistical surveys (of some 17,000 people) enquiring into their sexual behaviours. His particular areas of interest were the sexual responses of men, homosexuality, prostitution and premarital sex on college campuses. Kinsey agreed with Ellis' view of homosexuality as a normal variation of human sexual development and developed the idea of a continuum of sexual behaviour and proposed the theory that there were no homosexual, heterosexual or bisexual people, only acts (Hawkes 1996). Bisexuality, therefore, was a statistical combination of the numbers of heterosexual and homosexual acts any individual might have experienced. This approach has been criticised because it ignores the obvious reality that people do label themselves and others.

The work of Masters and Johnson follows on from that of Kinsey from the late 1950s to the 1970s. Masters was a gynaecologist (and Johnson his research assistant) and their work began by studying the physiological and anatomical aspects of female sexual responses. Unlike any of the other sex researchers (before or since), Masters and Johnson did direct observational work in their laboratories. Later, their work focused on sexual dysfunctions in married couples and, later still, they moved the focus of their work to homosexuality. Although much of the focus in Masters and Johnson's earlier work was on women's sexual responses and their work was very influential in highlighting the greater orgasmic capacities of women compared to men, they too have been the subject of much criticism by feminists.

Hite, the only woman to have worked independently on large-scale sexological research, conducted large-scale surveys of sexual behaviour in the 1970s. These took the form of written questionnaires, the majority of which were completed anonymously. Hite studied women's and men's sexuality separately. A staggering 100,000 questionnaires were distributed to women, of which 3019 were returned and analysed (Hite 1976), and 119,000 questionnaires were distributed to men, of which 7239 were returned and analysed (Hite 1981). In the report on women's sexuality there was an emphasis on women's experience of masturbation, orgasm and women's sexual experiences with men. There is also a very short section on lesbian sexuality. Hite argues that her emphasis on the more physical side of women's sexuality, in particular what arouses women to orgasm, was necessary as 'this has been so little understood and so long suppressed' (1981, p.xiii). By contrast, in her report on male sexuality she argues that the stimulation necessary for male orgasm is generally well understood and, therefore, her emphasis in this report was on how men feel about their sexuality and personal relationships (particularly with women) and whether they were happy and satisfied with their sexual lives.

Feminist critiques of sexology

There is a well-documented feminist critique both of sexology itself and of the major influential sexologists, whose work I have briefly outlined above. Both the theoretical perspectives and practical aspects of sexological research have been criticised, as well as the damaging consequences of it for women. Although a number of feminists have written on this subject, it is radical feminists, most notably Jackson (1983, 1984, 1987, 1994), who have produced the most extensive critiques.

Feminists have challenged the central tenet of sexology – that is, that it is a neutral and objective search for, and presentation of, the 'truth' about sex. This has been an important challenge for, as a twentieth-century science, sexology has had a legitimacy and status that has made its findings very influential, particularly with regards to women's sexuality. As Jackson has so clearly documented, sexology was just as biased and subjective as any other branch of scientific enquiry, if not more so (1984, 1994). What came to be presented and accepted as scientific facts were, in fact, reworked and strengthened versions of patriarchal myths about male and female sexuality which feminists had long campaigned to destroy. Not only was the content of this sexological work inherently anti-feminist but the timing and contexts of some of the most influential sexological research – for example, Ellis' work in the early twentieth century – was produced against the background of, and acted as part of the backlash to, active feminist campaigning on sexual matters.

All the major sexologists – Ellis, Kinsey and the Masters and Johnson team – have been criticised for similar reasons but there are also criticisms of their specific pieces of work. Taking the general criticisms first, all the sexologists have been accused by feminist writers of holding an essentialist model of sexuality with heterosexuality taken as the (absolute) norm. Despite attempts by all the sexologists not to pathologise and stigmatise homosexuality and bisexuality, these still have been clearly marginalised. Also, within heterosexuality, vaginal intercourse is given an absolute and inviolable priority – this has been called the 'coital imperative' (Jackson 1984, p.44). All other kinds of sexual activity are essentially regarded as preliminary (hence 'foreplay'), optional extras or substitutes for times when vaginal intercourse was not possible for whatever reason.

The second feminist criticism common to all sexologists is that they take 'as given, the particular form of male sexuality that exists under male supremacy and attempt[s] to universalise it, so that it becomes the model of sexuality in general' (Jackson 1984, p.45). Under this model – in which there is a total belief in the existence of a sex drive or instinct – sexual energy builds up over time and must be released one way or another. Allowance is made for individuals to have different amounts of sexual energy and men are generally thought to have more than women. Individuals, especially men, are not thought to have full control over their sexual urges, a belief which leads quickly to the removing of responsibility from men for acts of sexual abuse and exploitation, coincidentally – or, rather, not coincidentally – one of the main focuses of the feminist struggle, both historically and still today.

It is Ellis' work in particular which has been criticised for turning men's sexual violence towards women into an activity that was legitimate, normal and to be expected (Jackson 1994; Jeffreys 1990). He claimed that females of the human and all animal species were biologically programmed to show resistance to males' sexual advances but that they did not really mean their show of resistance for they wanted the males to 'conquer' them. Men were biologically programmed to do this conquering, for which the use of force was, if not always actually necessary, then certainly desirable. The experience of physical pain was considered by Ellis to be an integral part of women's sexual pleasure:

> Whilst in men it is possible to trace a tendency to inflict pain, or the simulacrum of pain on the women they love, it is still easier to trace in women a delight in experiencing physical pain when inflicted by a lover, and an eagerness to accept subjection to his will. Such a tendency is certainly normal. (1936, p.89)

It is not difficult to see why feminists now, and then, resented Ellis' reputation as a pro-feminist champion of women's rights. Although Ellis did support some rights for women, feminists such as Jeffreys have argued that his version of feminism was 'simply a glorification of motherhood and a development of the different but equal ideology' (1990, p.17). Ellis was strongly opposed to radical and militant feminists of his own time, especially the Pankhursts and the Women's Social and Political Union.

Kinsey's sexological work has been criticised by feminists for the way in which he trivialises the extent and nature of sexual abuse against women and children (Segal 1994). For example, he was of the opinion that teenage girls would commonly 'cry rape' in order to avoid getting into trouble with their parents for staying out late. With regards to the sexual abuse of girls by adult men, his intention appeared to be to gain his readers' sympathy for the men accused of these offences and to seriously underplay the effects of such abuse on the children concerned: 'in most instances the reported fright was nearer to the level that children will show when they see insects, spiders, or objects against which they have been adversely conditioned' (1953, p.121). As well as trivialising child sexual abuse in this way, evidence has emerged very recently that much of the 'data' on children's sexual responses was in fact supplied to Kinsey by the men who were sexually abusing them (Tate 1998).

Another feminist criticism directed specifically at Kinsey is that far from being a scientifically objective observer of human sexual behaviour, his work reveals that he was, in fact, deeply biased. As Dworkin (1981) has pointed out, despite the thousands of people he interviewed about their sexual behaviour, Kinsey claims not to have uncovered any instances of marital rape or any other abuse of women by their husbands. Yet he did manage to find and report 'several instances of wives who have murdered their husbands because they insisted on mouth-genital contacts' (Kinsey, Pomeroy and Martin 1948, p.578). Presenting such a biased picture of marital relations would be laughable in the 1990s but it is hard to believe that even in the late 1940s these could have been accepted as valid research findings.

Masters and Johnson have been criticised by feminists not only for the sexological research they did but most of all for the use to which they put their findings. Unlike the other sexologists, Masters and Johnson directly applied their findings to the development of what came to be known as 'sex therapy'. The theory and practice of their model of sex therapy has been hugely influential and still remains so with some sex therapists and psycho-sexual counsellors today. Feminists have argued that the whole basis of Masters and Johnson's work, especially the development of the Human Sexual Response Cycle (HSRC) model, 'favors men's sexual interests over those of women' (Tiefer 1995, p.55). Masters and Johnson began their research by interviewing prostitutes. Their rationale for this was that prostitutes were excellent informants on sexual response patterns because they had vast numbers of sexual partners and could sexually satisfy them very quickly (Brecher 1972). Masters and Johnson ignored any political dimension to prostitution and instead effectively gave female clients in their sex therapy the role of prostitute, whereby the women were clearly expected to service male sexuality. Thus their women clients were explicitly taught that it was their role to treat and cure any sexual dysfunction in their male partners, such as premature ejaculation. However, any sexual difficulties experienced by the women themselves were not serviced or treated by the men. Masters and Johnson also provided female sexual surrogate partners for their male clients as part of their therapy. There is uncertainty as to whether these surrogates were paid to have sex with the men – Jeffreys (1990) claims they were not paid but Szasz (1980) claims they were. Either way, it is clear that their job was to provide a sexual service to the men. Masters and Johnson, however, did not provide sexual surrogates for their female clients (Hawkes 1996). It is this blatant double standard to which feminists have drawn attention.

Jackson (1984) has described the principal aim of Masters and Johnson's work as being to cement heterosexuality and marriage through the maintenance of coitus at all costs. McNeil (1980) has described the aim of the Masters and Johnson sex therapy model as 'to help him get it up, keep it up, and ejaculate into the vagina: to help her open up and enjoy it' (p.47). This is a rather crude description but my reading of Masters and Johnson, and, indeed, of all the traditional sexology, suggests it is none the less an accurate one. That it was the aim of sexology and sex therapy to strengthen the heterosexual marriage bond can be of little doubt. However, curiously few of the feminists who have subsequently written on the subject venture any opinion on whether the aim was met or not. Segal (1987) is a notable exception and she is clear the aim was not met:

> If we are to accept, as indeed we might, that the conscious goal of Masters and Johnson's sex therapy, and that for which they were originally funded, was to shore up heterosexuality and marriage (and thereby male domination) by forging a bond of pleasure between the sexes, we have to conclude that they have spectacularly failed. The divorce rate has soared by 400 per cent in Britain over the two decades in which the sex therapists have supposedly fought to preserve marriage, even more in the US. It seems plausible to me, and the moral right would agree, that women's expectations of sexual pleasure (so often frustrated in marriage) are more likely to threaten than stabilize marital harmony, at least once women have any possibilities for economic independence. (p.98)

Returning now to the lack of feminist criticism of Hite's work, it is interesting to note that despite the fact that Hite has conducted her work from a more woman-centred and overtly feminist perspective than any other more traditional sexologists, her work seems to have been largely ignored by feminist observers. I have only been able to find one or two extended critiques of her work: Segal (1983, 1994) and Stanley (1995). Feminist books exclusively devoted to sexuality issues in which one might expect to find some reference to Hite's work omit it entirely – for example, Jeffreys' (1990) *Anticlimax* and Feminist Review's (1987) *Sexuality: A Reader* both have numerous references to Ellis, Kinsey and Masters and Johnson in their indices but Hite is not listed in either of them. Dworkin (1987) makes a brief reference to Hite's research to quote one of her findings (that most women do not orgasm through intercourse) and clearly rates Hite's work highly, describing her as 'the strongest feminist and most honorable philosopher among sex researchers' (p.148). However, Dworkin does not engage in any real discussion of Hite's work. Stanley (1995), in her book on sex surveys, has produced the most extensive critique of Hite's work that I have come across. She praises Hite's research for letting women speak in their own voices, on their own terms, about things that matter to them in relation to sexuality. Stanley highlights some methodological shortcomings in Hite's work, predominantly those relating to a lack of attention to epistemological issues and a lack of reflexivity – that is, Hite's failure to reflect on her own role as researcher.

However, Stanley also feels that Hite's work has methodological strengths, for which she has not received sufficient credit: 'The methodological innovation in Hite's work is its removal of "the numbers" from rhetorical and textual centrality, resulting in "a survey" that is different in form and function from the dominant post-war version of what this should be' (1995, p.230).

Segal (1983) is less positive than Stanley and criticises Hite's report on female sexuality for being too similar to Masters and Johnson, for focusing too heavily on what makes women orgasm and ignoring the social dimensions to women's sexuality, specifically failing to make links between sex and culture and sex and gender. Over a decade later, Segal argued that far from living up to its claims of offering a 'new perspective on female sexuality, which [stands] prevailing theory on its head' (Spender 1993, preface), Hite's work does precisely the opposite – that is, it reflects the limitations of the sexological tradition. Segal develops her argument that Hite views sex as a biological or purely physical experience and in so doing fails to take into account the social meanings which accompany the bodily experiences. In addition, Segal believes that Hite, in common with all other sexologists, is unable to theorise sexual desire. As Segal believes the complexities and contradictions of sexual desire are essential factors for investigation and understanding of sexual behaviour, it is not then surprising that she finds Hite's work somewhat lacking in insight (1994).

In another work Segal criticises not Hite's sexological research referred to in the previous section but her other large-scale survey *Women and Love*. Segal's criticisms again refer to Hite's lack of attention and sensitivity to social aspects of sexuality – that is, how race and class impinge on women's feelings and possibilities regarding personal relationships. She also comments on Hite's 'methodological mayhem' (1990, p.277). I would certainly agree with Segal on this latter point and feel that Hite has failed to successfully merge qualitative and quantitative methods and it is surprising that Stanley (1995) does not draw more attention to this in her critique. In my view, the results of Hite's work are unsatisfactory on a number of levels and I suggest that this is one reason why so little attention has been paid to Hite's sexological research: her findings are presented in a form that is very tedious to read. For example, with regards to the report on women's sexuality, the vast majority of the 664 pages are used to reproduce direct quotes from the women who completed the questionnaires. Many of these quotes say the same thing over and over again. Hite justifies her use of direct quotes in the following way:

...the Hite Report methodology was conceived as providing a large forum in which women could speak out freely – giving everyone reading those replies the chance to decide for themselves how they felt about the answers. The methodology was seen as a process, both for the individual women answering the questionnaire, and for the person reading what the 3019 women had written – a process of rethinking, self-discovery, and of getting acquainted with many other women in a way that had never before been possible – an anonymous and powerful communication from all the women who answered to all the women of the world. (1981, p.1059)

I agree with this to an extent – it is interesting and important to include women's own voices (and I have done it myself in this book). Nevertheless, this method of presenting research findings does seem somewhat overdone in Hite's work – for example, 15 pages of direct quotes from women whose masturbation fell into the type 1A category (see Hite 1976, p.79 for descriptions of the different types of masturbation). Obviously, Hite's readers could skip several pages at a time if they did not want to read all of her respondents' quotes, so I feel a more valid criticism is that it is very difficult to extract useful information from the presentation of the research findings. Occasionally there are precise percentage figures, which are easily retrievable and helpful – for example, 82 per cent of respondents said they masturbated and 15 per cent said they did not. However, at other times, actual numbers are given instead of percentages – for example, 80 out of 1844 women said unequivocally that there was physical discomfort during intercourse and 237 said unequivocally that there was not. At other times no figures at all were given and findings are presented in the form of 'the overwhelming majority of women' or 'many, many women'. Most annoying of all were the times when the reader was left with no idea of the frequency of women's responses to a particular question. Prior to reading the work, I was especially interested in Hite's findings about women's feelings regarding oral sex on a man (as this would have been a useful comparison to my own findings regarding women with learning disabilities). However, Hite presents her findings to the research questions 'Do you enjoy fellatio? To orgasm?' (p.374) merely as a set of 15 direct quotes (a mixture of positive and negative comments). There is no accompanying commentary, analysis or explanation of how representative or otherwise these 15 women were of the 3019 who replied to the survey or even whether the remaining 3004 had answered that particular question or not. In her report on male sexuality, which was produced some years later, Hite does seem to have improved the presentation of her findings. The vast majority of the 1129 pages are still filled with direct quotes but this time many of the research findings are given as percentages and, therefore, information can be more easily retrieved.

A major piece of British sex research was published by Wellings *et al.* in 1994. However, this work was concerned with providing data on what people did sexually and not with what they thought and felt about their own experiences or sexuality issues more broadly. The reasons for this are because the survey was located firmly within a framework of concern about sexual health and sought to provide data 'that would help in assessing and preventing the future spread of HIV' (1994, p.5). Although relevant in that sense, it has nevertheless been strongly criticised for what it did not investigate:

> The clitoris is not mentioned, let alone 'defined' anywhere in this research and nor is the occurrence of orgasm or sexual pleasure more widely in either women or men. Desire and pleasure are absent, along with consent and force, lust and pain, sorrow and joy...There are numbers and percentages aplenty, but little awareness that what gives life to these is how people understand and feel about what they do and do not do; research that excludes this, in my view, will not be able to explain very much of anything. (Stanley 1995, p.52)

The point was made earlier that sexology is often not merely descriptive but also prescriptive. A good example of this in recent years is Quilliam's *Women on Sex* (1994). Here, as well as reporting her research findings, the author provides a great deal of commentary to accompany the statistics and quotes. The author chooses to describe her respondents' answers by completely aligning herself with them and using the first person plural, hence 'we feel...' or 'we are more likely...'. At times she aligns herself so strongly with her respondents that it simply does not make grammatical sense. She mixes the first person plural with the single article, resulting in the bizarre phrases 'our clitoris' (p.135) and 'our husband' (p.202).

The book is written from a perspective that seems indiscriminately positive about women's sexual activity with men. Of course, there is nothing intrinsically wrong with presenting a positive picture of women's sexual lives – indeed it would be very welcome, if it were accurate. But the fact that the findings of this piece of research conflict with much of the other research in the area, combined with the lack of analysis of gender power relations, inevitably leads one to cast doubt on them. For example, the author does not draw attention to some of the more glaring inconsistencies in the women's replies, despite claiming that a cross-check for inconsistencies and exaggerations was done ('we found almost none' p.240). However, there clearly *are* inconsistencies: on the one hand, we are given to believe that almost 75 per cent of women share equally with men the role of initiating sex and that men almost always respond positively to these overtures (p.113) and yet, on the other hand, we are also asked to believe that 68.5 per cent of the women want more sex than they are getting (p.196).

Neither the author nor the respondents write within a framework that shows any gendered, political understanding of sexual relations between men and women. For example, in the discussion on women posing for their male partners to take sexual photos/videos (45.7% of the women had done this) there was not only a total absence of any analysis of why it is men photographing women and *never* the other way round but no mention of the possibility or actuality of women being pressured by their partners to do this. In addition, readers are, in fact, invited to understand and indeed excuse the men's abuse of the women's trust in this matter (by showing the pictures to their friends without the women's permission or knowledge): 'They constantly ask us to pose, loving to capture our beauty, and sometimes so proud of it that they take things a little too far' (p.176).

Vance (1983), observing sex researchers attending a conference, described them thus: 'Many were not just [sexual] enthusiasts, but missionaries and proselytizers' (p.379). The research described above is a prime example of this.

Feminism and sexuality

With the development of the Women's Liberation Movement and feminist thinking in the 1970s, traditional ideas about the nature of both female and male sexuality came under scrutiny. Challenging and changing ideas about sexuality as an abstract concept and sexual practice itself were central to feminism. In fact, it could be argued that sexuality was *the* issue for feminists in the 1970s: the 1978 National Women's Liberation Conference in Birmingham passed the motion to make 'the right to define our own sexuality' the overriding demand of the movement, taking precedence over all other demands. However, as Segal has pointed out, this was only achieved with such fierce debate and opposition that it effectively prevented any further National Conferences from being called (1987, p.96). Feminist preoccupation with sexual matters has a much longer history. Women had mobilised around such issues as the need to change sexual relations between men and women and rejecting male control over female sexuality as early as the 1880s (Jeffreys 1984, p.22).

Despite there no longer being any clearly defined women's liberation movement, sexuality is still a central concern for many feminists, although the nature of the concern, the analysis of the problem and the direction of proposed changes varies widely. The calls for women's right to sexual pleasure and fulfilment and to control our own bodies, which were central concerns in the 1970s, are rarely heard so directly today. This is partly because, for some women, some of these demands have been met and progress has undeniably been made. Instead, the debates today are more likely to be about which ways of achieving sexual pleasure are compatible or incompatible with feminist principles (e.g. the lesbian S/M debate, see Jeffreys 1994), whether pornography does or does not contribute directly to women's oppression (Segal and McIntosh 1992; Itzin 1994) or establishing the true extent of sexual violence (Kelly 1988). Some feminists regret this change from a positive call for women's sexual liberation in the 1970s to a negative and 'bleak sexual conservatism' in the 1990s (Segal 1994, p.xii). Others, whose work is rooted in what some see as the 'doom and gloom' school, argue that their work reflects the very real, and sadly, negative sexual experiences of many women (Holland 1992; McCarthy 1994). How representative women who have negative sexual experiences are of all women is not, and is unlikely ever to be, known and care needs to be taken in suggesting otherwise. However, feminists who try to promote a more positive view of (hetero)sexuality could just as easily be accused of overlooking the point of accurate representation or taking a simplistic view of it. For example, Segal (1994) quotes statistics from quantitative sexual surveys in the 1970s and 1980s showing how many women were happy with their sex lives with men. She suggests that the feminist magazine *Spare Rib* collapsed because young women were not impressed by the 'puritanism' of feminists. (Although this may have been a contributory factor, there were undoubtedly others, such as conflicts around race and ethnicity and wider economic factors which led to the collapse of not only *Spare Rib* but also a number of other women's collectives, most notably the *Sisterwrite* bookshop collective.) In trying to promote a sex-positive culture, feminists can make as many simplistic and sweeping statements as they accuse their sex-negative peers of doing.

To understand how feminists reached their current divergent stances on sexuality, it is necessary to examine contemporary women's responses to the sexual liberation era of the 1960s and to women's liberation in the 1970s. These processes have been charted thoroughly and differently by Jeffreys (1990) and Segal (1994), amongst others, so it is not necessary to do so again here. However, I will briefly examine some of the major feminist challenges to traditional ideas about sexuality.

First, feminists emphasised that sex was not a purely private matter between the individuals concerned. It was also a public matter because it was regulated by the law, medicine, religion and ideology. Feminists argued that the social context of sex must be understood, that there were clear patterns of sexual behaviour which could be observed and analysed. Having much in common with the sexual script theories of Gagnon and Simon I outlined earlier, Jackson (1978) stated unequivocally that 'sexual behaviour is social behaviour' (p.2). Until feminist sociologists like Jackson made it clear that sexuality could be investigated or understood only in its social context, sociologists had tended, if they had looked at it at all, to examine sexuality in isolation, taking it as a 'given' unproblematic entity.

Feminists placed gender into the centre of questions around sexuality and in so doing removed what had previously been considered all-important, namely object choice and deviancy. Thus it was argued then, as it still is now, that there are more similarities in the sexualities of gay and heterosexual (or straight) men or lesbian and straight women than between men and women. However, in recent years this position has been challenged by 'queer' theorists and activists who argue the opposite – that is, that there are, in fact, many similarities in the desires, identities and experiences of lesbians and gay men. Smyth (1992) describes queer politics as both an expression of lesbian and gay anger at the more overt and heightened oppressive measures adopted in the 1980s – for example, homophobic responses to the AIDS crisis, Clause 28 of the Local Government Act 1988 and as a backlash against what some perceived as assimilationist lifestyles and strategies of many lesbians and gay men. Far from arguing that they are just the same as heterosexuals, save for their same-sex desires, queer theorists seek to celebrate their difference.

In some of the early challenges to traditional views on sexuality, feminists argued that the concept of sexuality and, in particular, ideas about sexual practices were male defined. As I explained earlier in relation to sexology, sexual activity was largely viewed in terms of penetration (real sex). Anything else (not real sex) was considered merely a preliminary to penetration or as a substitute for it. Sexual language reflected this with a multitude of words and phrases to describe intercourse and a paucity of terms to describe other sexual acts. Active verbs describing men's role in sex and passive verbs describing women's role were, and are, standard. The role of the clitoris in women's sexual pleasure was emphasised by feminists and most women's real sexual experience – that is, of clitoral, rather than vaginal, orgasms was explained (Koedt 1970; Hite 1976). Some of the most important feminist criticisms related to the nature of male sexuality in particular. The commonly held notions that men had greater sexual appetites than women and that they had a right and a need to satisfy their appetites were vigorously challenged. This challenge led to a huge shift in awareness of, and responses to, male sexual violence, which is covered in more detail below.

The challenge to the belief in the naturally larger sexual appetites and 'promiscuity' of men also led to challenges in traditional thinking about prostitution and the dichotomy between good and bad women. The traditional view had it that it was necessary to have a 'pool' of 'bad' women to service the sexual needs of men as this prevented 'good' women from having to meet those demands. The 'bad' women thus provided a protective service. Feminists challenged the assumptions behind this thinking (Jeffreys 1985). One of the most important feminist contributions to understanding male sexuality was to try to expose the myth of men's supposed lack of control over their sexual response. It was, and still is to some extent, believed by both men and women that men have only limited sexual control and that they can be sexually aroused with little or no warning. Women were considered responsible for men's sexual arousal, not by saying or doing anything in particular but simply by being there: 'The male has a semi-automatic response set which seems only minimally related to any particular female' (Stewart 1981, p.167). Although this sounds faintly amusing, one only has to think of the deadly serious effect such thinking has had on women's dress codes, whether in Victorian Britain or some Islamic cultures, today. Feminists challenged the assumption that women were responsible for men's sexual arousal and satisfaction, not least because women were also held responsible for their own (which meant that men were responsible for neither). Traditionally, women were expected to enjoy what men enjoyed and blamed and subjected to 'treatment' if they did not. Men were not expected to change their sexual practices to suit women. These glaring double standards were exposed and challenged by feminist theorists and activists.

Another major area of feminist criticism related to women's right to control their own fertility. The social prohibitions on having a child outside marriage are easy to forget for most women in Britain today, now that they have largely disappeared. But these prohibitions were very real in the (not-so-distant) past and still are very real for women from certain religious and ethnic communities. These strong social prohibitions and the lack of adequate contraception and abortion facilities have historically conspired to force women to regulate their own, and men's, sexual desires for fear of the consequences.

One of the major contributions of lesbian feminists to the sexuality debates was to challenge not only the supposed superiority of hetero-sexuality but, equally important, to challenge its taken-for-granted status. Instead of accepting the traditional view – held by some feminists as well as non-feminists it must be said – that heterosexuality was *the* natural form of sexuality, lesbian feminists exposed some of the pressures on women to be heterosexual (Rich 1980). These pressures vary from subtle forms of ideology to the not so subtle economic pressures or even direct physical force (Jackson 1987).

Other major contributions to the sexuality debates come from black feminists, who have been critical of white feminists for failing to understand the complex inter-relatedness between sexism, racism and class oppression. White feminists have identified with their victimisation as women and so have privileged the fight against sexism as *the* struggle. In doing so, white feminists have inadvertently overlooked or deliberately ignored the advantages that racism grants them as white people (Hill Collins 1991). This lack of appreciation of how, in particular, racism and sexism work together to oppress Black women has led to white feminists asking absurd questions of Black women about whether being Black is more important than being a woman (hooks 1984).

Some of the major campaigns of the early second-wave feminists were so clearly from a white middle-class perspective that it is not surprising that many Black women felt alienated from them. Some of these related to sexuality and others did not – for instance, Friedan's (1963) emphasis on women's need and right to work outside the home makes sense in the context of white, middle-class, college-educated women who felt they were wasting their education and intellectual abilities but did not speak to the experience of poor Black women who had always worked outside the home as a matter of economic necessity and whose history was a cruel one of enforced and exploited labour; similarly, whilst white feminists were understandably campaigning for the right to control their own fertility through access to contraception and abortion, few gave voice to many Black women's concerns about racist ideologies which worked to prevent them from having children (Mama 1986). The cultural specificity of much of Western feminism's response to issues of sexuality is also to be found in its response to the problem of sexual violence (see below for further discussion).

Despite its inevitable shortcomings, the effect of feminism on traditional views of sexuality was nevertheless radical and transforming, turning long-held beliefs on their head and firmly placing a fair share of responsibility for their behaviour and ideas with men. Nowhere was this more obviously the case than with the whole issue of sexual violence.

Feminism and sexual violence

Many of the first-wave feminists in the late nineteenth century had campaigned around issues of men's sexual use and abuse of women (Bland 1995). However, as Jeffreys (1984) points out, their efforts have largely been forgotten or are now viewed as conservative or retrogressive because of their associations with the ideas of social and sexual purity. Nevertheless, it is the case that women like Josephine Butler (who campaigned to challenge men's use of prostitutes and their sexual abuse of children), Millicent Fawcett (who, with regards to incest, argued that men who so abused their position of trust should receive an especially harsh punishment) and Elizabeth Wolstenholme Elmy (who campaigned for the law to allow women to be able to refuse sexual intercourse with their husbands) and many others like them were actively debating ideas and organising political campaigns on issues which are still very much alive in the late twentieth century.

Of the second-wave feminists, it was Griffin, with her paper *Rape: The All American Crime* (1971) and Brownmiller, with her book *Against Our Will: Men, Women and Rape* (1975), who are widely credited with beginning the current wave of exposing the nature and extent of men's sexual violence to women. Feminists have done much over the past twenty or so years to increase understanding of sexual violence. One of the most important achievements has been to dispel many of the myths that surrounded the issue. By doing this through academic research, use of anecdotal evidence, through women's groups and conferences, but, perhaps more importantly (because it reaches a bigger audience), through television, radio, women's magazines and newspapers, the truth about sexual violence has started to emerge. This, in turn, gives more women the confidence to speak out, which, in its turn, helps to build a clearer picture of what really happens. Thus more women are believed (Plummer 1995).

Amongst the most important of the myths that feminists have helped to dispel are: that women enjoy sexual violence; that women provoke it by their behaviour and/or appearance; that women routinely make false accusations about it; that it only happens to certain kinds of women; that the most common form of sexual violence is a disturbed man raping an unknown woman in a dark alley at night. A full exploration of these myths and the feminist challenges to them have been adequately conducted elsewhere (e.g. Kelly 1988; London Rape Crisis Centre 1988), so it is unnecessary to do so again. Instead, I want to emphasise how feminists have focused on the vitally important task of placing the responsibility for the continued existence of widespread sexual violence with men individually and collectively. Whereas traditionally women had been partly or wholly blamed for their own violations, from the 1970s onwards this was vigorously challenged. Thus feminists refused to accept terms and concepts like 'dysfunctional' or 'incestuous families' and, instead, substituted terms such as 'father–daughter rape' (Ward 1984). In doing so, an accurate description of the dynamics of the situation is offered and the responsibility is removed from the whole family to the individual perpetrator. This was important because the beliefs that are held about men, women and rape do not just have an impact at the theoretical level. Rather, they have policy and practice implications: what a society believes about sexual violence determines the kind of services and support structures that a society will provide for those affected.

Especially important has been the feminist challenge to the public/private split that existed not only in the minds of individual men and women but was, and still is, enshrined in the responses of statutory agencies and the legal system. The traditional view on this was that, first, what happened behind closed doors, at home, was of concern primarily to those involved and, second, where it was brought to public attention it was, by definition, treated as less serious than any comparable 'public' crime and attracted a lesser penalty, sometimes no penalty at all. The fact that rape within marriage was only criminalised in England and Wales in 1991 (one year earlier in Scotland) and that there still have been only a handful of successful prosecutions is the most obvious manifestation of this. Similarly, it is largely because of this public/private split that if a man rapes an unknown child, he will not only be treated as a criminal but often vilified as the worst kind of will not only be treated as a criminal but often vilified as the worst kind of criminal. Yet if another man rapes his own child (bearing in mind that there is every likelihood the rape will be repeated many times as opposed to the likely 'one-off' rape of an unknown child), he may well not be treated as a criminal at all but diverted towards therapy (Kelly 1988; Radford and Stanko 1996).

With regards to sexual violence perpetrated towards adult women, there is a strongly held belief that it is, quite simply, worse to be raped by someone you do not know than someone you do. I myself was involved in a very public exchange of views on this issue in the pages of *The Observer* newspaper in 1992. In response to the highly publicised conviction of the American boxer Mike Tyson for raping a woman he knew, journalist Simon Hoggart had categorically stated that being raped by a stranger was a worse experience for women (16.2.92). The newspaper printed my response, which argued that this belief stems from the wholly false assumption that rape is essentially to do with sex and, therefore, is not so bad if it is by someone you know. I challenged Hoggart to produce some evidence for his claims – that is, accounts from women who had been raped by acquaintances, friends, boyfriends, etc, who said it was not so bad (23.2.92). None was ever produced. MacKinnon, on the other hand, has produced a very well-argued challenge to the traditional public/private split and has proposed that legally there should be no such distinction because: 'when women are segregated in private, one at a time, a law of privacy will tend to protect the right of men to be let alone, to oppress us one at a time... It will keep some men out of the bedrooms of other men' (1987, p.148).

Feminists have gone to great lengths to demonstrate that the over-whelming majority of perpetrators of sexual violence are men (Kelly 1996) and that men of all classes, occupations, ages and races can commit such offences. Nevertheless, the use of gender-neutral language to describe the perpetrators of sexual violence is deeply ingrained in our culture and efforts to shift from this position are strongly resisted (Randall and Haskell 1995). A good example of this is highlighted by Campbell (1988) in *Unofficial Secrets*, her book on the Cleveland child sexual abuse scandal of 1987. Anal dilatation had been one of the key diagnostic factors of this 'epidemic' of child sexual abuse (and, certainly, in media reports it was this diagnosis that was focused on to the exclusion of all others). It was accepted by all who believed that the children had been penetrated that they had been penetrated by penises – this was based on the children's own accounts. Nevertheless, throughout the emerging scandal and the subsequent inquiry the vast majority of those involved consistently referred to 'parents' as the alleged abusers/wrongly accused, rather than fathers. Of this phenomenon, Campbell wrote:

> It became the unsayable thing during the inquiry. It was almost as if a society which was finally being forced to confront child sexual abuse was at the same moment refusing to confront the character of the perpetrators and the sexual system which produced abuse. And although the modern women's movement, like its antecedents in the late nineteenth and early twentieth centuries, has been among those who brought sexual abuse out of the shadows, and has certainly focused on masculinity as a political problem, it was exiled from the national debate surrounding Cleveland. (1988, p.63)

I would argue that for many people it is still largely unsayable today and using gender neutral terms when discussing learning disabled perpetrators of sexual abuse is quite common. An example from the mid-1990s was a research grant proposal which was returned by the funding body for amendment because its title specifically said it was to investigate the difficult and abusive sexual behaviour of *men* with learning disabilities. The title was duly changed to say people with learning disabilities but the proposal itself, and the work, was, in fact, solely investigating men's sexual behaviour. The funders had no objection to this and recognised the need for it and funded the work but it seemed that they were unable to openly and publicly confront the issue head on. The reasons for this are unknown but could possibly include wanting to 'tone down' the gendered political dimension to the work and also because they wanted to be seen to be leaving open the possibility of women as perpetrators of sexual abuse. Whilst it is, of course, the case that women can, and do, sexually abuse others, this specific piece of research was not concerned with that and was only looking at the sexually abusive behaviour of men. However, it must also be said that there are also prominent researchers and practitioners in the learning disability field who feel it is 'wholly inaccurate and unhelpful' to use gender neutral terms and who caution against it (Thompson, Clare and Brown 1997, p.16).

Another of feminism's most important contributions to promoting the understanding of sexual violence has been to highlight the connections between different types of sexual violence (e.g. rape of adult women, sexual abuse of children), sexual aggression (e.g. sexual harassment, indecent exposure, obscene telephone calls) and other forms of violence against these connections and puts forward a very sound case for looking at men's behaviour and women's experiences in the context of a 'continuum of sexual violence' (p.27). If we add to the phenomena Kelly describes such things as men's use of pornography, their use of prostitutes (both male and female) and the hitherto largely unrecognised ways men use their power sexually over other men (Jones 1991; Thompson 1994), it is hard to avoid the conclusion that sexual aggression and violence are integral parts of how masculinity and male sexuality are constructed under patriarchy.

However, not all feminists would fully support that argument. Segal (1990) argues that 'it is less than helpful, however, to tie up all forms of aggression, sexual violence, institutionalised heterosexuality, warfare and ecological destruction in one neat package as "male"'. She continues:

> In sifting through the growing literature on men's coerciveness and abuse of women, I suggest that it *is* possible to make distinctions: between men who deploy violence against women and men who do not; between one form of violence and another; and between the structures which foster and maintain different forms of violence and those which help to undermine them. (p.xiii)

Other criticisms levelled at the way feminists have viewed the links between sexual violence and masculinity concern the lack of adequate theorising of the sexual violence perpetrated by women, whether that takes the form of child sexual abuse or sexual abuse within adult relationships, both heterosexual and lesbian. There is no doubt that these are under-researched and poorly understood phenomena by feminists and non-feminists alike. However, some work is being done to examine the phenomenon of women's violent behaviour, both sexual (e.g. Elliot 1993) and physical (e.g. Lobel 1986), and it is hoped that understanding will develop in time. Kelly's work (1996) has made an important contribution to this.

Black feminists have also criticised the white feminist response to the phenomenon of sexual violence for again failing to understand how racism impacts upon it. This manifests itself most obviously, but not exclusively, in the racist myth of the archetypal rapist being a Black man raping a white woman. The legacy of this myth is that Black women have not traditionally joined feminist campaigns to fight sexual violence: '...if black women are conspicuously absent from the ranks of the anti-rape movement today, it is, in large part, their way of protesting the movement's posture of indifference toward the frame-up rape charge as an incitement to racist aggression' (Davis 1978, p.25).

toward the frame-up rape charge as an incitement to racist aggression' (Davis 1978, p.25).

This leaves Black women very vulnerable in their communities, however, as most Black women are raped by Black men. In seeking to protect individuals and/or communities from oppressive intrusions by a white racist police and legal system, Black women 'live with the untenable position of putting up with abusive Black men in defence of an elusive Black unity' (Hill Collins 1991, p.179). Consequently, some Black commentators have been critical of violent Black men's reliance on, and exploitation of, Black women's community loyalty (Mama 1989). However, this is not only an issue that affects women because of their race and racism. It can be an equally strong pressure on women because of their religious or political beliefs. Women from the republican community in Northern Ireland have vividly described the same tension in their lack of reporting of sexual and domestic violence by republican men. They summarise the situation thus: 'It is contradictory to expect women to phone the police for support in areas where the dominant community perception of the police is of repression rather than one of support' (McKiernan and McWilliams 1994, p.15). Just as the police in Northern Ireland may use the reason for being called to help a republican woman as an excuse to search for signs of membership of the IRA, so white police in Britain, on being summoned to help Black women who are experiencing violence in their homes, may 'turn the whole affair into an immigration investigation' (Mama 1989, p.17).

Conclusion

This chapter demonstrates that, despite its shortcomings in theory and practice, the achievement of feminism in developing insights into issues of sexuality and sexual violence has been considerable. What first-wave feminists had begun in the late nineteenth century, the second-wave feminists finally succeeded in doing in the 1970s and 1980s. This achievement was to 'name' aspects of women's sexual experiences and feelings that had not previously been named and, therefore, could not be spoken about. If, as I will later clearly demonstrate in this book, women with learning disabilities are getting a raw deal in their sexual relationships with men, it is entirely thanks to feminist efforts that we can, first, recognise that this is the case; second, understand why it is the case; and, third, see how the situation might be transformed.

CHAPTER TWO

Learning Disability – Ideologies and Sexuality

Amidst all the changes in ideology and principles of care, definitions and labels, and theories about causation and treatability of the condition, only one thing has been constant: the presence of people with learning disabilities in society. From the earliest recorded history, people with learning disabilities have been a source of speculation, fear, pity or curiosity for others. They have usually been set apart from other people, often literally, and the feelings they have aroused in others have rarely been positive. In short, by their very existence, people with learning disabilities have posed a challenge to the rest of society.

An early Christian belief saw 'fools' – as they were usually referred to – as being closer to God than ordinary people, due to their simplicity of mind and uncorrupted nature; they were so-called 'holy innocents'. This contrasted sharply with another strongly held early Christian belief of fools being possessed by the devil. There are records of people with learning disabilities being tortured and killed as witches during the Inquisition (Hattersley *et al.* 1987). It is generally accepted that up until the Industrial Revolution, when most people would have earned their living off the land and from home-based activities, that having a family member with a learning disability would not necessarily have been a particular burden. In pre-industrial societies, including some contemporary ones, there were relatively few people with profound or multiple disabilities as they tended to die from complications associated with their condition and/or they may have been actively or passively killed off. (If this sounds inhumane, we need remind ourselves that in the world's most 'advanced' societies people with learning disabilities are still 'allowed to die' by necessary medical treatments being withheld (Sobsey 1994) or are prevented via genetic screening from being born in the first place (Thompson 1993).) Historically, people with less severe learning disabilities may have been able to contribute to family life and income by carrying out simple, but necessary, tasks and, as work was home-based, there would have been other people present to provide the necessary supervision for those who needed it.

During and after the Industrial Revolution, when the labour force became more controlled, structured and urbanised in factories, it is easy to see the impact this would have had on people with learning disabilities: with the profit-driven emphasis on quick and efficient production in factories, they were unlikely to be able to contribute and, as work was no longer home-based, there may have been no one to look after them. For those who were now a drain on the family's resources, a solution to the harsh choices of locking them in the home or putting them out on the streets to fend for themselves began to present itself: the emergence of the institution; 'Social historians have shown that institutional life was practically unknown in pre-industrial society' (Laslett 1965, p.11). However, in the early nineteenth century there was a rapid development of public institutions, not only for people with learning disabilities but also for the old, the sick, the mentally ill, the criminal, etc.

As well as the direct effect of the Industrial Revolution, a philosophical movement also played its part. From the 1780s to the mid-nineteenth century in a number of Western European countries, it was the so-called Age of Reason and Rationality. As a consequence, it was thought appropriate and necessary by some to observe and analyse the 'mad' or 'subnormal', to make sense of their behaviour. In order to do this they had to be in a place where they could be observed. Institutions, or asylums as they were more commonly known, were ideal for containment and observation. Indeed, they are still used today for that very purpose.

Although they became, and largely remain to this day, repressive and dehumanising environments, it is important to recognise that the intentions behind the early institutions were benevolent: they were seen as model environments (Tuke 1813). But, however good the intentions, with hindsight it is clear they were not realised. The reasons for this are varied and complex but it has been suggested that the demise was related to both the growth in the numbers of institutions themselves and the numbers of people in them (Scull 1979). The reasons for the phenomenal growth are complex and varied but include a failure to live up to expectations of being able to cure patients and return them to their communities combined with an ever-expanding definition of who could be classified as 'mad'. It is important to note at this point that although I am attempting to give some historical context to the treatment of people with learning disabilities, the early asylums did not clearly distinguish between with learning disabilities and those with mental health problems. Like other institutions – for example, workhouses and prisons – they took a mixture of young and old, men and women, and, in the terminology of the time, both imbeciles and lunatics. As Scull (1993) describes it, 'the asylums were largely receptacles for the confinement of the impossible, the inconvenient and the inept' (p.370). Another reason for the expansion of institutions was an ever-increasing public demand for the service, although, as Scull (1993) has so meticulously researched and documented 'it was the existence and expansion of the asylum system which created the increased demand for its own services, rather than the other way around' (p.363).

However, it was not merely because of practical problems associated with growth that the institutions did not live up to their developers' hopes. The theoretical basis to their work also became corrupted. The 'moral management', with its emphasis on will-power, obedience and conformity, became in itself a rigid discipline which destroyed people's individuality (Ryan and Thomas 1987).

Another significant historical development was the medicalisation of the condition and its treatment. The early proponents of institutions were lay reformers and educationalists and the institutions were run by lay superintendents. But doctors became concerned that a whole field of work was slipping away from them and they successfully campaigned for more control, eventually taking charge of the institutions and their inhabitants. This shift towards the medicalisation of what had hitherto been considered essentially a *social* problem was to have a profound effect on the way people with learning disabilities were viewed and treated. Only towards the end of the twentieth century could one say that the medical power base has begun to diminish. It has been my recent experience that within the remaining institutions it is still the doctors who are very much in control of what happens to individuals with learning disabilities, despite the fact that services as a whole are managed by non-medical staff.

Because of the influence of the medical profession, the prevailing ideology, until very recently, has been to define people with learning disabilities in terms of what is wrong with *them*. Their 'deficiencies' and their 'subnormality' have been emphasised and little attention has traditionally been paid to the negative way they have been treated by society and what effect this has had on their lives and opportunities.

However, in recent years ideologies and services have changed and the social model of disability has been increasingly influential in the learning disability field. Therefore, attention is more and more being paid to the effect society has had on people with learning disabilities. Consequently, the labels attached to people with learning disabilities have also undergone much revision over time. In what they call the 'client terminology cycle', Dunne and McLoone (1988) argue most convincingly that merely changing the label does little or nothing to change people's social identity. If the social status of a group remains the same – that is, marginalised and oppressed – then the new label will inevitably become debased in time: 'Breaking the client terminology cycle requires not only a change of words, but also such fundamental social changes as will ensure that those who have been marginalised become valued members of the community' (p.61). This is undoubtedly the case – neither the women's movement, the gay liberation movement, the Black civil rights movement or any emancipatory struggle has ever argued merely for an improvement in the labels used to describe them. There has always been an awareness of how language is used as an instrument of oppression but the demands for change have always gone beyond terminology.

Normalisation

In the past two decades there have been two major changes in the ideology affecting services for people with learning disabilities: first, the adoption of the principles of normalisation, which have had an enormous impact; and, second, the growth of the self-advocacy movement, where the effect on services has not been so great to date but which, nevertheless, is having a steady and growing impact.

Normalisation as a concept originated first in Denmark and took hold in Scandinavia in the late 1960s and early 1970s. The definition, which is widely credited as being the first, is 'to create an existence for the mentally retarded as close to normal living conditions as possible' (Bank-Mikkelsen 1980, p.56). Ideas about normalisation as a set of specific concepts for learning disability services were framed by a wider recognition of the human and civil rights of people with learning disabilities – in 1971 the United

Nations issued their *Declaration of General and Special Rights of the Mentally Handicapped*, the first statement of which was that people with learning disabilities should have the same basic rights as other citizens of the same country and of the same age. The early Scandinavian ideas on normalisation (Bank-Mikkelsen 1980; Nirje 1980) went on to be developed in North America (Wolfensberger 1972, 1983). In Britain, O'Brien's work has also been influential. Through the development of what are known as the 'Five Accomplishments' – that is, presence, choice, competence, respect and participation – O'Brien has usefully drawn out the practical implications of normalisation for people with learning disabilities (Emerson 1992).

The fact that practically every service for people with learning disabilities has adopted at least some of the principles and practices of normalisation (and those which have not are likely to keep quiet about it) is a testament to the strength of the ideology. This is not to say, however, that the concept is unproblematic. Most common criticisms focus on the way that normalisation, at times, obscures, and, at times, rides roughshod over, equal opportunity issues. In relation to race and ethnicity, these have been well analysed by Baxter *et al.* (1990) and Ferns (1992).

There is also a developing body of feminist criticism of normalisation. Writers such as Brown and Smith (1989, 1992) argue that there are many similarities between the oppression of people with learning disabilities and the oppression of women. They suggest that there are also theoretical parallels between the solutions offered by feminism for women's emancipation and those offered by normalisation for people with learning disabilities. In practice, however, there is some divergence – for example, normalisation advocates small-scale services serving small numbers of people, who are not encouraged to have much to do with each other. As feminists, Brown and Smith have argued, this can lead to problems being individualised and commonalities and patterns overlooked. The social and political context of people's lives is then poorly understood. Similarly, normalisation promotes the ideal model of residential services as the small group home for, and staffed by, both men and women – essentially replicating a 'family home' (Burns 1993; Clements, Clare and Ezelle 1995). The predominance of this model takes little account of much feminist research, which has shown that in such settings women tend to bear a disproportionate amount of domestic responsibilities (Rose 1982) and that living in isolated family units can be dangerous for women and children

(Barrett and McIntosh 1982; Campbell 1983). The value of communal support and protection can be overlooked in normalisation.

Normalisation strongly promotes the idea that individuals with learning disabilities should mix (socially, educationally, at work) with non-disabled people. Once again, it overlooks the value many women (or Black people, or gay men and lesbians) place on 'self-segregation' or separatism as a way of gaining confidence and of feeling relaxed away from the dominance and gaze of those who oppress them. The more recent development of the self-advocacy movement, which, as I will outline below, is based on a sense of shared identity and solidarity *amongst* people with learning disabilities, flies in the face of this particular principle of normalisation. There is a world of difference between choosing to associate primarily or exclusively with those like oneself and effectively being forced to, as has been the case for so long with people with learning disabilities. In seeking to overcome the negative sides of past services, normalisation principles can sometimes advocate things, such as primarily associating with non-disabled people, which can amount to throwing the baby out with the bath water.

In highlighting the recent critiques of normalisation I am in no way suggesting that the whole ideology is worthless. It has been immensely valuable in improving the lives of millions of people with learning disabilities. Nevertheless, it is a flawed concept and, therefore, needs critical analysis, and crucially anti-discriminatory practice needs to be built into its implementation. Without an underlying valuing of, and respect for, difference, the tendency will inevitably be towards changing people with learning disabilities into what society wants them to be instead of valuing them for who they are.

Self-advocacy

If normalisation is based on the premise that it is society which handicaps people by the limited and devalued experiences it offers and that the way to overcome this is to increase people's social status, it follows that individuals should be given a say in the way they live their lives. Self-advocacy is the obvious vehicle for this. As with the normalisation movement itself, the history of organised self-advocacy can be traced back to Scandinavia (Sweden specifically) in the late 1960s. It gained momentum in North America in the 1970s and established a firm hold in Britain in the 1980s.

Self-advocacy has a number of meanings and operates on a personal and political level. Individuals voicing their opinions about the day service they are offered, a users' committee liaising with the day centre management team and representatives of people with learning disabilities on social services department planning committees are all examples of self-advocacy. Essentially, the term refers to people speaking up for themselves and on behalf of others and, as such, clearly does not only apply to people with learning disabilities. (Citizen advocacy refers to non-disabled people acting as advocates for people with learning disabilities, usually on an individual basis.) Some individuals with learning disabilities may be naturally assertive, know what they want and not be shy about coming forward. Others may need structured and systematic teaching and support to understand the concept of 'rights' to be able to communicate effectively with others and to be able to operate in a group (Williams and Shoultz 1982).

In Britain today the national organisation called *People First* is run by a small group of people with learning disabilities with help from non-disabled supporters. It exists to provide information, support and training to other people with learning disabilities and staff in services. In addition there are numerous small and local self-advocacy groups as well as several other larger and well known groups across the country – such as *Advocacy In Action* in Nottingham and *Skills For People* in Newcastle – which perform largely the same functions. Many day services, especially Adult Training Centres or Social Education Centres, have user committees. (See Simons 1992 for details on the types, and impact, of self-advocacy groups.)

Self-advocates have produced information and training packs (see, for example, Brindley *et al.* 1994; Skills For People 1994). People with learning disabilities are increasingly being asked to act as consultants to academic teaching courses, research projects and the media. On the more creative side, people with learning disabilities are occasionally to be found on the stage or on television as actors – although, it must be said, only in 'disability arts groups' or when the part is specifically that of a learning disabled character. Some people with learning disabilities are also finding their voice in matters of social policy that go beyond learning disability services but which, nevertheless, affect their lives – for example, expressing their opinions on how the law should treat them when they have been the victims of crime (Williams 1995); or people with Down's Syndrome expressing their views on the plastic surgery conducted on children, or the abortion of foetuses, with their condition (Young People First 1994).

Despite its many achievements and the irreversible nature of the development (it is hard to imagine that any service provider is going to say in the future: 'we've changed our minds, we don't think service users' views are important after all'), the self-advocacy movement has not had anything like the same impact on services as the normalisation movement. This is because although normalisation meant a radical re-shaping of services, it did not fundamentally alter the power base – non-disabled people were still left in charge of the direction services should and would take and there was, and still is, an attitude of 'we know best'. For example, the voices of (albeit the minority of) people with learning disabilities who said they would prefer to stay in hospitals were drowned out by non-disabled converts to normalisation, who put that down to their being institutionalised and not knowing what community care had to offer. That may well be the case, but the fact remains that their voices were not heard and it is an example of how two philosophies which do go very well together can, nevertheless, sometimes conflict.

Learning disability services have still not yet fully grasped the nettle of genuine service user involvement in all aspects of service planning and delivery. Their tardiness in this matter is not a reflection on the lack of ability of people with learning disabilities to contribute in this way: the development of the Powerhouse (see p.77) is an outstanding example of how women with learning disabilities were involved at every stage of a complex planning operation. Rather, the reluctance of services to fully take on board the need for empowerment and self-advocacy has been due to the usual reluctance of those in power to relinquish it. To acknowledge that people with learning disabilities have an important part to play in the development of services can be seen by some service providers as an erosion of their professional skills and training. In short, it can be perceived as a threat and, therefore, resisted. This may work at a sub-conscious level; at any rate it is rarely openly acknowledged and discussed. Certainly, some professionals do voice criticisms of the way self-advocacy is practised but these are usually weak and do not stand up to rigorous scrutiny – for example, a common criticism is that the movement is dominated by the more able and articulate people with learning disabilities. This is certainly the case but it is also the case for practically any other emancipatory movement and, to a large extent, is inevitable – the most able are always going to have an advantage over the less able, certainly as far as the more visible side of the work – such as public speaking and direct action – are concerned. Self-advocacy is also criticised for not being democratic enough, that it is, in effect, a few individuals purporting to represent a large number of other people. Again, this is true but far from unique to the self-advocacy movement:

> When it comes to the challenge of self-advocacy, it seems the 'able' world can develop a scrupulous concern for the ideals of democracy – forgetting, perhaps, that in any community democracy means that a few politically active people represent the majority who are not politically active at all. (Shearer 1986, p.179)

Another important reason why some services have been slow to take up some of the challenges of self-advocacy relates to weighing up its obvious advantages with some of its less obvious disadvantages. The downside of both the theory and the practice of empowering service users to speak up for themselves and, where necessary, challenge service providers is rarely put. However, such a critique is needed, otherwise there is a danger that the rhetoric of empowerment can act as a smokescreen to hide the very real vulnerability of some people. As yet, no respectful replacement for the old paternalistic approach of 'looking after' people has emerged (Brown, personal communication). An example of this from the field of sexuality and learning disability is the stance taken by a leading self-advocate and peer educator on the issue of learning disability services producing sexuality guidelines. He felt that such guidelines should not be produced as other, 'ordinary', people did not have guidelines written about their sexuality (Brown, personal communication). This is partly true, although one could argue that laws and social norms regarding sexual behaviour act as guidelines in themselves. Also, such an argument overlooks the fact that such guidelines are not there primarily to regulate the sexuality of people with learning disabilities but rather to ensure a respectful and consistent response to individuals by staff and managers in services.

Some self-advocates with learning disabilities, particularly those who have public profiles at conferences and in the media, seem not to recognise that as people with mild learning disabilities who live relatively independent lives, they may have little in common with people with much more severe learning disabilities who are highly dependent on others for all aspects of their personal care and development. An example of this attitude is seen in a 1994 television programme on self-advocacy in which the following statement was made:

> The difference between mild learning difficulty and severe learning difficulty is less than most people would think. We all come from the same background, we came from separated schools...but we have the

same rights, whatever our disability is to speak for ourselves and learn the skills to do that. (Bull 1994)

Such a view, in my opinion, masks the very significant and special needs of less able people. Their real inability to make sophisticated judgements about their sexuality (or, indeed, about anything) may be overlooked by some of the more able self-advocates in their understandable drive to claim the right to be treated the same as everybody else in society.

Deinstitutionalisation

As I have outlined above, the growth of large institutions continued throughout the nineteenth and twentieth centuries, reaching a peak of some 64,600 people with learning disabilities in hospitals in the mid-1960s (Bone, Spain and Fox 1972). It was in the late 1950s and early 1960s that dissatisfaction with institutions began to surface publicly. Interestingly, the earliest dissatisfactions were registered in the legal field, rather than the medical, psychological or social work fields – in 1951 a National Council for Civil Liberties (NCCL) report, *50,000 Outside the Law,* drew attention to the lack of legal safeguards in the detention of people with learning disabilities in hospitals and highlighted the fact that hospitals had a vested interest in retaining patients rather than releasing them (Korman and Glennerster 1990); and in 1957 the Royal Commission on the law relating to mental illness and mental deficiency contained what is widely regarded as the first reference to community care (Renshaw *et al.* 1988). Despite the fact that ideas about the undesirability of institutionalised care were forming in the late 1950s, it was only some twenty years later that actual hospital closures were contemplated and some forty years later the process of deinstitutionalisation is still far from complete. The latest government figures available indicate that in 1997–98 in England alone there were approximately 6300 adults with learning disabilities still in hospital, the majority of whom were long-stay residents (Dept. of Health 1998).

During the 1960s and 1970s there were several influential publications which contributed to public and professional awareness that institutions were inappropriate places of care. Goffman's (1961) work on asylums introduced the concept of the 'total institution' and demonstrated its damaging effects on its inhabitants. General studies of the poor conditions of mental handicap hospitals, such as Morris (1969), and more specific inquiries into allegations of ill-treatment and appalling conditions, such as the Ely Hospital Report (DHSS 1969), contributed to the drive to consider whether hospitals could ever be suitable places for long-term care. It is important to note that reports and criticisms of mental handicap hospitals did not appear in isolation. Rather, they were part of a growing awareness of the negative effects of institutionalisation on other people too – for example, the elderly (Townsend 1962; Robb 1967). The 1971 White Paper, *Better Services for the Mentally Handicapped*, and the 1979 Jay Report on mental handicap nursing and care, both recommended running down hospitals and developing community-based services.

As well as the changes in policy prompted by humanitarian concern for the people who received the services and a belief that people's behaviour and symptoms could be successfully managed in the community by use of medication, there can be no doubt that economic factors played their part in deinstitutionalisation. Indeed, some commentators argue that money was *the* deciding factor (Korman and Glennerster 1990).

The arguments against hospital care and for community-based services have largely been won. Lone voices, such as that of Rescare (an organisation largely of parents of people with learning disabilities which campaigns for the retention of institutions, albeit in the form, some would say guise, of 'village communities') are not credited with much authority or influence by professionals in the learning disability field (Collins 1997). The fact is that most of the hospitals which are not already closed are actively working towards that end. However, a note of caution needs to be sounded here as some commentators (see, for example, Collins 1995) argue very convincingly that some of the more recent developments, such as learning disability hospitals becoming NHS Trusts, are working against the deinstitutionalisation process.

Concerns have, of course, been expressed about the kinds of community services that are replacing hospitals. As community implicitly, and sometimes explicitly, means families and families usually means women, there were many fears that the impact of community care would mean a significant increase in women's unpaid caring responsibilities (Dalley 1988; Finch and Groves 1983). However, my own involvement in, and knowledge of, people with learning disabilities being resettled from hospitals into the community suggests that the overwhelming majority do not return to live with their families but, rather, move into staffed provision in the statutory, voluntary or private sector. Research evidence confirms this (Donnelly *et al.* 1994).

It is not my intention to go into depth on the topic of deinstitutionalisation as that has been done elsewhere, including international comparisons (Mansell and Ericcson 1996). However, it is important to note that evaluating the success or failure of community care services is no easy task and is often not even attempted on a formal basis. However, the need to do so seems strong, for, as history shows, reforms which were initially well intentioned can inadvertently turn into repression, given the right conditions (Ryan and Thomas 1987). When we take into account the fact that research now shows that community care is *not*, in fact, cheaper than hospital care (Cambridge *et al*. 1994; Emerson, McGill and Mansell 1994), it is not beyond the realms of possibility that some might start to argue for abandoning it and rebuilding hospitals.

One of the most thorough evaluations of community care for people with learning disabilities is that carried out by the Personal Social Services Research Unit (PSSRU) at the University of Kent one year and five years after resettlement (Cambridge *et al*. 1994; Knapp *et al*. 1992; Renshaw *et al*. 1988). (Further research is currently being conducted some ten years on; see Cambridge *et al*. 1996.) Generally speaking, most of the improvements in people's lives and skills were made during the first year after leaving hospital and little or none in the subsequent four years (Cambridge *et al*. 1994, 1996). Although this may seem on one level somewhat disappointing, in fact it would be wrong to judge such findings at face value. In terms of individual satisfaction, most people were happier in the community than in hospital. Taking people's own, sometimes very long, histories of disadvantage and discrimination into account, there should be no reason to expect them to 'improve' after a mere five-year period and certainly no reason to even contemplate whether it is 'worth' resettling people from hospital into the community. After all, living in the community alongside everyone else is not just about attaining certain skills or behaving in a certain way. As the authors of the study themselves state:

> Beyond quality of life outcomes and individual abilities lies the central issue of human rights. Every one should have the right to develop their full potential and to experience life to the fullest...Ordinary, everyday experiences are harder to achieve in hospital than in community settings. (Cambridge *et al*. 1994, p.105)

Learning disability and sexuality

Historical perspectives

In order to understand how the sexuality of people with learning disabilities is viewed today, it is necessary to understand how it was viewed historically.

As soon as a historical view is taken, it is apparent that strong stereotypes prevailed. The first of these was the stereotype of people with learning disabilities as being 'eternal children'. Because of their limited intellectual capacity, people with learning disabilities were considered to forever have the mind of a child. They were associated with child-like interests and pursuits and often treated as if they were children (Craft and Craft 1983; Kempton 1972). In contrast to this image was the other stereotype of people with learning disabilities as being potentially dangerous. This was based on the idea that they were unable to control themselves and historically it had sometimes also been believed that they possessed a 'super-human' strength, so they could not easily be controlled by others (Hattersley *et al.* 1987).

If these were the general views held about people with learning disabilities, views about their sexuality, or lack of it, fitted into those distorted frameworks. Within the 'eternal child' context, people with learning disabilities were thought quite simply not to be sexual beings. As children were once considered to be asexual (this idea itself has undergone much revision; see Wyatt, Newcomb and Riederle 1993), people with learning disabilities, if they were just overgrown children, must also be asexual. Whilst this belief was held, any signs of sexual interest or arousal were ignored, repressed or misunderstood. In addition, and this is a crucially important point for understanding how sexuality issues for people with learning disabilities are managed or mismanaged today, it was thought essential to keep them in a state of ignorance about sex. Just as it was unthinkable to talk to young children about sex, so it was unthinkable to talk to adults with learning disabilities about sex – protecting their natural innocence was the priority and this fitted into an 'ignorance is bliss' philosophy. Within the belief system that saw people with learning disabilities as potentially dangerous, the effect this had on ideas about their sexuality are clear: it was thought that people with learning disabilities would have an uncontrolled sexuality, that they would be 'over-sexed', sexually promiscuous. In short, they were thought to be a potential sexual threat to others (Koegel and Whitmore 1983).

In summary, then, we can see that with the first set of beliefs it was people with learning disabilities who needed to be protected from all the sex that was going on in society; and in the second set of beliefs it was society that needed to be protected from all the sex that people with learning disabilities had within them. It is, of course, the case that these two belief systems are inherently contradictory, as Craft (1987) has observed. However, that did not stop them from both becoming very powerfully held 'truths' which exerted a powerful influence over attitudes to, and services for, people with learning disabilities. The legacy of those beliefs can still be observed today.

Another belief system which it is vital to understand because of the devastating impact it had upon the lives of people with learning disabilities is the eugenics movement of the late nineteenth and early twentieth centuries. Amongst others, people with learning disabilities were thought to be a threat to the 'stock of the nation'. Fears grew that the national heritage of intelligence and ability was being eroded by those at the lower end of the social scale. It was primarily women with learning disabilities, labelled then as 'feeble-minded', who were thought to be promiscuous, immoral and likely to produce large numbers of children similar to themselves (Kempton and Kahn 1991; Rosen 1972). Because the national gene pool was thought to be at risk, action was considered necessary to stop such 'unfit' people from reproducing. The strategy to prevent people with learning disabilities (as well as people with epilepsy and people with some physical disabilities) from reproducing had two main approaches: one was the continued use and further development of isolated institutions where the sexes were segregated – which I have already described – and the other, which was adopted more in the USA than Britain, was the introduction of compulsory sterilisation laws (Barker 1983). Sterilisation was thought to be a desirable option because:

> it is better for all the world, if instead of waiting to execute degenerate offspring for crimes, or to let them starve for their imbecility, society can prevent those who are manifestly unfit from continuing their kind. The principle that sustains compulsory vaccination is broad enough to cover cutting the fallopian tubes... Three generations of imbeciles is enough. (Buck v. Bell, 1927)

Although there were people with learning disabilities who were sterilized in Britain, the concentration in this country was on institutionalisation. However, it was thought advisable to use both tactics – that is, institutionalising people so that they could be 'trained and socialised', then 'voluntarily' sterilising them with a view to reestablishing them back in their own communities (Blacker 1950).

Within the large institutions people with learning disabilities were segregated from the rest of society and the sexes were strictly segregated from each other (Potts and Fido 1991). Although this segregation of the sexes was clearly to prevent any heterosexual activity and, most importantly, to prevent reproduction, it was also, initially, on grounds of propriety. For example, in the nineteenth century, the Commissioners in Lunacy complained when they discovered that an asylum mortuary contained corpses of both sexes; 'an arrangement, we think, objectionable' (1871, p.131).

It is important to note that the 'treatments' of institutionalisation and sterilisation were imposed not only on people whom we would recognise now as having a learning disability. The 1913 Mental Deficiency Act created a new category of person, that of the 'moral defective'. Moral defectives were thought to be those who might be sexually vulnerable, sexually promiscuous or who might behave inappropriately in public. A large proportion were, in fact, women who had illegitimate babies and who had nowhere else to go (Potts and Fido 1991). In addition to this was the fact that for an unmarried woman to have given birth to a baby without the means or ability to maintain it was in itself grounds for certification as 'feeble-minded' under the 1913 Act. This certification was for life, although subject to a five-year review. I have myself worked with a number of older women who were sent to mental handicap hospitals because they had had children or for, as they themselves described it, 'going with the men'. Some thirty or forty years later they were still there. Many of the people who were originally sent to hospitals as moral defectives or 'feeble-minded' may never have had a learning disability at all. However, after a whole lifetime of institutionalisation they are often indistinguishable, at least superficially, from those who do.

Given that society once had such a negative and stigmatising attitude towards the sexuality of people with learning disabilities, we need to understand both that things have changed considerably for the better and why the changes have happened.

Contemporary perspectives

In contrast to the past, it would be unusual now to find many people who have significant contact with people with learning disabilities who would deny that they have sexual feelings or rights. There is evidence to suggest that parents of people with learning disabilities tend to find it more difficult to accept their sons' and daughters' sexuality than professional carers do (Rose 1990; Squire 1989). The reasons for this undoubtedly vary but include the fact that parents obviously have a much greater emotional bond with their children than professionals do with their clients, and this leads, amongst other things, to parents tending to take a much more longer term view of the issues than professionals. Priorities for consideration and action sometimes also differ between parents and professionals (Rose and Jones 1994). However, the stereotypes of parents of people with learning disabilities as being completely unapproachable and refusing to discuss sexual matters are largely myths (Brown 1987; Ryan 1993). As Craft (1983a) has pointed out, 'parents generally are not good at helping their children achieve psycho-sexual maturity. Many a child gets there *in spite of* rather than *because of* parents' (p.4, original emphasis). Parents of people with learning disabilities, therefore, should not be judged any more harshly than other parents if they do not wholly welcome signs of developing sexuality in their daughters and sons.

Professionals, who, as I have outlined above, were at the forefront of the repressive measures taken to deny people with learning disabilities their rights to sexual expression in the nineteenth and twentieth centuries, have, on the whole, undergone a considerable shift in attitude and professional practice. Although negative attitudes persist amongst significant numbers of staff working in learning disability services (Johnson and Davies 1989), most accept the sexual needs of their clients. The essential issue for today's service providers is no longer one of complete denial and repression of their clients' sexuality but the management of it (McCarthy 1991). However, before I outline how sexuality issues are managed in learning disability services today, it is necessary to examine what prompted such a huge shift in attitude.

There are two separate, but connected, movements which are usually credited with having produced the change. These are, first, the development during the 1960s of a more liberal and open attitude towards sexual matters in society generally and, second, the adoption of principles of normalisation in learning disability services – which, as I have already explained, meant giving people the opportunity for as ordinary and 'normal' a life as possible. Opportunities for sexual expression, in theory at least, had to be included in this process.

However, there is a third factor which is not given prominence in the literature when the change in attitude and practice is discussed (e.g. Segal 1983; Van Zijerfeld 1987) but which I consider to be as influential as the first two factors, if not more so – namely, the widespread availability of effective contraception. The availability of, in particular, the contraceptive pill (which was not freely and overtly available to unmarried women in Britain until 1974) meant that for the first time in history, people with learning disabilities, like anyone else, could have sex without inevitably having children. Given the great fears about people with learning disabilities reproducing and the draconian lengths society and professionals were prepared to go to prevent this, one cannot but fail to see how important a role contraception has played in effecting change.

By looking at how attention has been paid to the sexuality of people with learning disabilities, we can see what the priority areas are and how these have changed over time. For example, a review of the relevant literature of the 1970s shows a clear emphasis on the right and need for sex education. Alongside this, and, indeed, within the suggested sex education curricula, was a strong bias on the themes of heterosexual dating and marriage. Wolfensberger (1972), whose beliefs about sexuality fit into the models which understand it as a strong biological urge, argued that it was simply not fair to expect certain groups in society to remain celibate. He saw sexual expression as a right, but only within certain limits: he saw the benefit of a heterosexual relationship as being so 'self-evident that it scarcely requires discussion' (1972, p.169). Despite advocating support only for heterosexual relationships, in a rather cryptic final paragraph he recognises that, given time, he might be able to advocate a broader range of possibilities. Like a number of others writing at this time (see below), he was convinced of the need for heterosexual couples to refrain from having children. He makes no mention of the vulnerability of people with learning disabilities to sexual abuse; indeed, he makes no mention whatsoever of anything remotely negative about sex at all.

Lee (1972) also argued for the right for people with learning disabilities to date the opposite sex and marry, again with the proviso that they 'should not be persuaded of their right to procreate' (p.9). Katz (undated but published in the same volume as Lee) makes exactly the same points. Once again, no mention is made of same-sex relationships nor of the potential for negative or abusive sexual experiences. The lack of attention to the negative side of sexual life is undoubtedly partly due to the lack of awareness at that time that people with learning disabilities could be abused. It is unfair to judge past works by today's standards. However, it is not entirely true that professionals always lacked this awareness: Lowes (1977), in describing the need for a sex education programme, mentions that some of the people with learning disabilities who were to attend had experienced incest, prostitution and exploitation by a more experienced partner. Nevertheless, the sex education that was subsequently offered to them focused on heterosexual dating, marriage, reproduction and childbirth and did not include matters concerning abuse or protection.

Some writers in the 1970s, however, did have a more realistic insight into the need for people with learning disabilities to be more fully prepared for their sexual lives. Kempton (1971) and Kempton, Bass and Gordon (1972) mention sexual vulnerability and suggest that it is wise to explicitly teach girls with learning disabilities that they do not have to have sex merely to please boys and to teach boys with learning disabilities that they should not be sexually aggressive. (It is a measure of how little things have changed in sexual relationships between men and women that, over a quarter of a century later, the exact same messages are still being given in sex education materials – see, for example, McCarthy and Thompson 1998.)

Greengross (1976) and Stewart (1979) both wrote similar books about sexuality for people with a wide range of disabilities which contained chapters on learning disability. Stewart follows the pattern I have described above in advocating teaching on marriage and reproduction but omitting references to sexual abuse and vulnerability. He makes a useful contribution to knowledge by highlighting that abnormal or inappropriate environments produce inappropriate behaviours, including sexual behaviours. He calls for a greater understanding of this phenomenon. Greengross acknowledges, in passing, that people with learning disabilities can be sexually exploited and puts the blame for this largely on the lack of sex education given to young people with learning disabilities. Curiously, the two examples she gives of the lack of sex education making people vulnerable relate to the onset of wet dreams and menstruation and have nothing to do with sexual exploitation. Like Wolfensberger, both Greengross and Stewart believe that sex is a biological necessity and that sexual relief is of paramount importance. Greengross advocates the use of pornography, vibrators, artificial penises, rubber dolls, sex surrogates and prostitutes to ensure that disabled people get their 'necessary' sexual relief. An illustration of how much thinking about sexuality in disability services has changed in the past two decades, can be seen in the way both Greengross and Stewart discuss sex between staff and clients. Although both recognise that it could be problematic, they are in favour of it in certain circumstances. Greengross describes staff who would be willing to do it (or indeed who have done it) as 'humane' (p.108) and 'compassionate' (p.109). Stewart declares that many staff 'must have been tempted towards it on the grounds of mercy alone' (p.102). The use of the word 'mercy', which is normally applied to alleviating desperate or extreme circumstances, does rather imply that not to be able to achieve sexual satisfaction causes great suffering and that staff should see it as part of their duty to relieve that suffering. Almost all sexuality policies and guidelines produced in the 1980s and 1990s (see, for example, East Sussex County Council (undated); Hertfordshire County Council Social Services Dept (1989)) clearly prohibit all sexual contact between staff and clients. This is in recognition of the vulnerability of people with learning disabilities to being abused by those with power and authority over them. (See below for a further discussion of sexual abuse.)

Also in the 1970s there were two major research studies on the marriages of people with learning disabilities, something which has not been done since. The fact that marriage did not continue to be an area for continued research interest may be due to the increasing acceptability for people generally, and also people with learning disabilities, to live together without marriage. However, it is also a reflection of the fact that despite the emphasis in early sex education on marriage, the reality was that it never materialised as a genuine option for the vast majority of people with learning disabilities, particularly those who rely on services to support them. Nevertheless, the two 1970s studies were important. Mattinson's (1970) study and that by Craft and Craft (1979) both depicted marriage as a predominantly positive choice and lifestyle for the couples they researched. Both studies emphasised the complimentary nature of the partnerships, which enabled the couple to function adequately or well as a unit, whereas each individual's limitations would probably have led to a less satisfactory outcome.

A disappointing feature of both these studies on marriage is the lack of analysis concerning the fact that there is a strong pattern of the husbands being intellectually more able than their wives. This is a phenomenon I have observed in my own social work and sex education practice and which I have drawn attention to in my writing (McCarthy 1996a). Mattinson (1970) makes the observation that it is a 'particular point of interest that the majority of husbands were more intelligent than their wives' (p.183) but she does not discuss the point further. Craft and Craft (1979) do not pay attention to the phenomenon, although the information that the husbands in their study were indeed generally intellectually more able than their wives is found in table 1a on p.40. We are told that some of the intellectually more able men had a mental illness or psychopathic disorder, but 12 of the 45 were 'normal' (p.40). Scally (1973), reporting his own findings in Northern Ireland and commenting on those of Mattinson, interprets the phenomenon of men being more able than their wives in the following way: 'We can logically assume that a mentally retarded girl can be more attractive to a man than a mentally retarded male would be to a female' (p.190). This is obviously true but still does not address the question *why*. My own view on this, based on my work experience, is that women with learning disabilities are often attracted by the higher social status of a non-disabled man (see also Chenoweth 1996) and that non-disabled men are attracted by the fact that they can dominate their partners and shape the relationship to meet their own needs.

The lack of a political gendered perspective on marriage and sexual behaviour is found in both books at various points. Mattinson, for example, relates a situation where a couple with learning disabilities argue and the wife locks the husband out of the house while she does her housework, telling him that he can come back in when his tea is ready. He then proceeds to attack her, kicking her in the face, cutting her eye, kicking her leg and bruising her spine. Mattinson describes this incident in the following way: 'This scene ...illustrates how the "victim" of domestic battles usually sets up and invites the violence and is as much of a protagonist as the partner who is finally charged with assault' (p.138). Because a week later the couple are reconciled and the woman appears to be affectionate to her husband, Mattinson describes this as proof of 'positive enjoyment of physical violence' (p.138). Such a naïve and unsympathetic interpretation would certainly not have been unusual at this point in time. The first refuge for women escaping violent men only opened in Britain in 1972 (Pizzey 1974) and the nature and extent of domestic violence only started to be properly understood once feminists and sociologists gave it the attention it deserved (see, for example, Dobash and Dobash 1980; Stanko 1985).

Although Craft and Craft do not overtly excuse abusive behaviour by the men they studied, they do, nevertheless, display a simplistic and generous view of it. For example, prior to marriage, 9 of the 45 husbands had convictions for rape and indecent assault (usually of children), with 6 of the 9 having several such convictions. After marriage, only 2 were re-convicted of similar offences. This is seen by Craft and Craft as a sign that 'sexually active men, who before marriage molested children ... afterwards had *little or no need to do so*' (1979, p.123, my emphasis). This implies that men need a sexual outlet and if a lawful one does not exist, they are compelled to find an unlawful one. Such attitudes were widely held, are clearly a product of their time and must be seen in that light. Neither should it be assumed that authors who once held such views do not change them as time passes and awareness increases – in the 1980s and 1990s Ann Craft, for example, went on to produce some of the most pioneering and influential work on sexual abuse and learning disability in this country and abroad.

Moving on to the 1980s, the first thing to observe is that the volume of literature increases enormously. If the topic of sexuality was first opened up in the 1970s, it was during the 1980s that it broadened and developed. Because of the volume of literature in the 1980s and, indeed, the 1990s (to date), I do not intend to systematically review all of it here but rather to give an overview of the issues it tackles and prioritises and to examine how these developed from the rather narrow concerns of the 1970s. In fact, in reviewing the 1980s literature it is clear that it is still the right and need for sex education which predominates as a theme. At this point in time, however, the literature presents us with many practical examples of how sex education can, and should, be put into practice (see, for example, Craft and Craft 1983; Robinson 1987; Thaler Green 1983). Reports of more detailed and specialised teaching on sexuality issues also emerge, such as teaching menstrual care to girls and women with learning disabilities (Demetral, Driessen and Goff 1983; Fraser and Ross 1986).

In recognition of the fact that professionals are not the only ones who influence and, indeed, to a large extent, control the sexual lives of people with learning disabilities, the literature also begins to emphasise the need to understand parents' perspectives (Fairbrother 1983) and the need for staff to work collaboratively with parents (Brown 1987; Stevens et al. 1988).

Reproductive rights, or lack thereof, also become a significant issue for debate within the literature in this decade. Examples of specialised contraceptive services for women with learning disabilities are given (e.g. Chamberlain et al. 1984). Within this particular strand of the literature the contraceptive options are discussed in a very 'neutral' tone, without the more 'political' analysis of the use, over-use and mis-use of contraception that would be offered in later years (e.g. McCarthy and Thompson 1992). The use of the injectable contraceptive Depo-Provera is a case in point here: during the 1980s it is suggested as a perfectly acceptable method of contraception, especially for those women with learning disabilities who were not thought reliable or motivated enough to take the Pill regularly (Committee on Drugs, cited in Chamberlain et al. 1984), but by the 1990s, with the benefit of hindsight regarding the side- and after-effects, as well as a gendered, political perspective on sexuality matters, it is suggested that use of Depo-Provera should be challenged as it 'is disproportionately used with women with learning difficulties, as well as other disadvantaged groups of women' (McCarthy and Thompson 1992, p.70). Contraceptive options for women with learning disabilities are discussed more fully in Chapters Four and Five.

However, it would certainly not be true to say that the controversial side of the debate about reproductive rights was totally undeveloped in the 1980s. The issue of sterilisation was a strong theme of the literature, particularly in 1987 and 1989 when there were two high-profile legal cases concerning the sterilization both of the under-18s – the 'Jeanette' case – and the over-18s – in *Re. F.* A number of topical papers appeared at that time outlining the moral and legal arguments surrounding sterilization without consent (Carson 1989; Roy and Roy 1988) and examining the alternatives (Davis 1987; Tonkin 1987). Reproductive rights in relation to parenting also begin to be a developing feature of the literature in the late 1980s. In contrast to the (what I have suggested elsewhere as misguided) emphasis on reproduction and looking after babies that was such a strong feature of much of the 1970s sex education for people with learning disabilities, the 1980s literature moves onto a different plane. Thus the plethora of negative myths about people with learning disabilities as parents are explored and largely dispelled (Tymchuk, Andron and Unger 1987), although the very real problems of social isolation, poverty, poor parenting models (Andron and Tymchuk 1987) and unsupportive or abusive male partners (Gath 1988) are not glossed over.

As well as actually providing sex education, assessing levels of sexual knowledge of people with learning disabilities is much written about during the 1980s (Bender *et al.* 1983; Brown 1980). Detailed checklists for assessing what information people with learning disabilities already had were provided (Craft 1983b), although some writers do point out the limitations of such exercises, namely that 'with the many inhibitions that surround sexuality, the information imparted may have little reference to the individual's true knowledge or attitude' (Leyin and Dicks 1987, p.143).

As well as the development of an academic and professional literature during the 1980s, there was also the development of staff training packs (e.g. Dixon 1986) and sex education materials especially designed for work with people with learning disabilities. Apart from Dixon's *Sexuality and Mental Handicap* (1988), which is a workbook with ideas for group exercises, the resources are almost always visual ones – the Craft slide packages (1980, 1985) and Kempton's *Life Horizon* slides (1988) being excellent examples. Craft's slides cover appropriate social behaviour, menstruation and reproduction, whilst Kempton's look at physical and sexual development, heterosexual relationships, sexual health issues, reproduction and appropriate and inappropriate sexual behaviour. The Kempton pack, despite the breadth and depth of the issues covered (there are approximately 1000 slides in the pack), pays only cursory attention to same-sex relationships. The Brook Advisory Centre's *Not a Child Any More* pack (1987) is an example of a different kind of visual resource: a work pack of pictures and discussion ideas accompanied by two large anatomically correct (almost correct, they do not have anuses) dolls. The dolls (one female, one male) and the pictures demonstrate yet again a strong heterosexual bias. It is not until the 1990s that this particular feature of sex education materials begins to change.

Because of the development of interest, skills and materials for supporting people with learning disabilities in their sexual lives during the 1980s, both statutory and voluntary services were obliged to 'legitimate' this new area of work through the adoption of formal policies and guidelines (see, for example, Dumfries and Galloway Social Work Dept. undated; Mencap Homes Foundation 1987). Within these, the organisational context for the work is made clear through the setting out of the principles, values and procedures each service expects its staff to adopt. (For a thorough examination of the issues concerning policy development, see Booth and Booth 1992; Fruin 1994; McCarthy and Thompson 1998.)

The expansion of literature on sexuality issues shows no sign of abating during the 1990s. Quite the opposite. More and more sex education materials have been produced and the academic and professional journals reflect the increasing level of interest in the field. In the 1990s the literature demonstrates how new strands of work developed, as well as how old themes were revisited and reworked.

Probably the most striking development in the 1990s is the way in which the real – that is, often uncomfortable and harsh – circumstances of people's sexual lives were confronted. Brown (1993) describes this a 'major paradigm shift' (p.623). Rather than the approach which had often been taken in the 1970s, which indirectly implied that people with learning disabilities could simply be educated into having the same kinds of sexual lives as other people, there was more of an emphasis on understanding and respecting difference – for example, of the assumption that people with learning disabilities are just the same as other people, Hingsburger and Ludwig (1992) contested that 'While this may be laudatory, it is also a mistake. People with disabilities have a vastly different life history than those without disabilities' (p.3). This is not to say, however, that despite their different and disadvantaged lives, many people with learning disabilities do not wish to be like other, non-disabled people. Indeed, the desire for that is strong in many people, a factor which has long been recognised (e.g. Edgerton 1967). In the 1990s it was further demonstrated how this wish could, in itself, further disadvantage people – for example, in order to be in a socially valued relationship, women with learning disabilities might be willing to accept sexist or abusive treatment from their partners (Burns 1993; McCarthy and Thompson 1992).

In seeking to ground sexuality work in the reality of people's lives, five major new strands of work have been developed in the 1990s: positive representations of same-sex relationships, awareness of gender power relations, the need for a multi-racial and multi-cultural approach to sexual matters, HIV prevention work and a greater understanding of the nature and extent of sexual abuse.

As I have made clear above, same-sex relationships were either ignored, marginalised or pathologised in the early sexuality literature. In the 1990s, however, sex education materials were produced which, for the first time, were genuinely from an equal opportunities perspective, presenting relationships and sex between women and between men as positive and valued (Lewisham Social Services 1992; McCarthy and Thompson 1992). In a way that seems unthinkable, certainly in the 1970s and even the 1980s, some writers are now very critical of homophobia in other people's work (e.g. Hingsburger and Ludwig 1992). The concept of institutional homosexuality (whereby all same-sex relationships were explained by the argument that people had no other choice and their natural heterosexual instincts were, therefore, 'perverted' by the circumstances in which they lived) was *very* prevalent in the early writings. In the 1990s it is now challenged, not because it has no validity – for some people in some circumstances it may be the most useful description of what is happening – but because it implies that same-sex relationships are, by definition, second best to opposite-sex ones (McCarthy and Thompson 1998; Thompson 1994b).

Sex education materials *are* still produced which marginalise same-sex relationships or which, underneath a veneer of acceptance, are still essentially homophobic. For example, Monat-Haller (1992), in answer to her own stark question 'Are same sex relationships harmful?', considers the possibility of a man with epilepsy biting off his partner's penis if a seizure were to occur during oral sex and the possibility of transmitting HIV or other sexually transmitted diseases. As these situations could just as easily be applied to heterosexual situations, there seems no obvious reason to consider them specifically in relation to same-sex activity – other than to try to present it as undesirable.

The reasons for the shift towards a more positive view of same-sex relationships are varied. I would suggest that the greater social acceptance of lesbians and gay men in some contexts in the 1990s, as compared to ten or twenty years ago, is a strong contributory factor. Amongst other things, this had led to more workers in learning disability services being 'out' at work. The personal agenda of key individuals in organisations can make a tremendous difference in creating a positive attitude towards homosexuality, even if the service as a whole and most of the people in it remain essentially homophobic (McCarthy and Thompson 1995). Clearly, HIV/AIDS has played its part too; the urgency of the need to provide good safer sex education, particularly to men with learning disabilities who have sex with men and the irresponsibility of not doing so, has in itself been partly responsible for the shift in attitude (Cambridge 1997; Thompson 1994a). (HIV issues are discussed more fully below.)

A gendered political perspective on the lives of, particularly, women with learning disabilities has also developed in recent years. This relates not only to directly sexual concerns but more generally to broader life experiences (Brown and Smith 1992; Burns 1993; Williams 1992). Some writers, myself included, have gone to great lengths to demonstrate that the gender power relations and gender conditioning which affect other people also affect people with learning disabilities too. Having worked with men and women with learning disabilities on matters relating to sexuality and sexual abuse, Simpson (1994) concluded the following:

> This distinction between women and men's experience, needs and ways of expressing them is an important aspect of people with learning difficulties' lives. What became very clear was the extent to which people with learning difficulties pick up gender conditioning. Although many of them are isolated and/or live segregated lives they do not escape gender conditioning. (p.16)

My own work with women with learning disabilities and that of my male colleagues on the Sex Education Team (now CONSENT) allowed us to see very clearly that women and men with similar ability and communication levels, living in the same environments, with the same staff teams, nevertheless experience their sexual lives in very different ways. My conclusion on this phenomenon is that, with regard to their sexual experiences, women and men with learning disabilities 'have more in common with their non-disabled counterparts than they do with each other' (McCarthy 1993, p.278). The research project documented in this book has been part of my ongoing exploration of this.

The reasons why this gendered analysis of the sexual lives of people with learning disabilities has developed are similar to the reasons I outlined above regarding the development of a positive attitude towards homosexuality: namely, a greater social acceptance of feminist ideas and practice than in previous decades, which has led to feminist women and supportive, non-sexist men (in the field of sexuality and learning disability these are predominantly gay men) feeling confident to put their political beliefs into practice at work. The fact that feminist ideas and writings have gained academic status and publishers know there is a large market for our work (Spender 1981) means it is now possible to get work published that previously may have been rejected as being too radical or of minority interest only.

The third of the new strands of sex education work in the 1990s is the awareness of the need to approach sexuality work in a way that fully incorporates the experiences of Black and ethnic minority people. This strand is the least developed (not least because there are relatively few Black people influential in the field) but awareness is certainly there now, where previously it was lacking. Sex education workers have come together to share ideas on how best to meet people's needs in a multi-cultural society (Landman 1994). Although it is relatively easy to ensure, for example, that Black and ethnic minority people are fully and positively represented in sex education materials (e.g. McCarthy and Thompson 1992), this does not mean that it always done (e.g. Craft *et al.* 1991). However, merely reproducing images of Black people is not a very sophisticated approach to the issue and certainly is not an adequate response (McCarthy and Thompson 1995). There is room for much improvement in this area. Baxter (1994) and Malhotra and Mellan (1996) have clearly outlined some of the factors which need to be taken into account when providing culturally appropriate sexuality support to people with learning disabilities from all backgrounds.

The fourth new development in sex education work in the late 1980s and 1990s was a focus on concerns around safer sex and HIV prevention. Unlike with the other more recent developments, the reasons for this one are stark and obvious in that HIV was only discovered in the early 1980s. Most of the HIV-related work has focused on the production of sex education materials specifically for people with learning disabilities (see, for example, McCarthy and Thompson 1992; O'Sullivan and Gillies 1993; West London Health Promotion 1994). Whilst this work on safer sex education is far from easy, it is, nevertheless, the most straightforward of the various strands of HIV-related work. Less attention has been paid to more complex areas such as the need for services to take on board the full extent of their protective responsibilities if people with learning disabilities are at risk and unable to protect themselves (McCarthy and Thompson 1994a; Thompson 1995). What is also often missing from the literature is a clear gendered perspective for doing HIV prevention work with people with learning disabilities which acknowledges the disadvantages women often face in seeking to negotiate and practice safer sex. Elsewhere, I have highlighted this weakness and offered suggestions for good practice (McCarthy 1994, 1997).

Although there is by no means a consensus, a strong voice has emerged within the learning disability field arguing that all HIV prevention work must prioritise the needs of men with learning disabilities who have sex with men. The reason for this is that, as with the general population in Britain, men who have sex with men continue to be at the highest risk (Cambridge 1997; Thompson 1994a).

Finally, another significant development in the 1990s, which will undoubtedly continue to grow, is the involvement of people with learning disabilities themselves in providing sex education and producing sex education materials. The organisation *People First* have had a sexuality officer who provides both peer education and staff training and examples are growing of visual (*People First* undated) and, particularly, video resources (South East London Health Promotion Service 1992; Walsall Women's Group 1994). Although there are one or two examples of this kind of work from the 1980s (e.g. the video *Between Ourselves* 1988) the development of peer education by people with learning disabilities has grown out of the self-advocacy movement I described earlier in this chapter. (See Chapter Six for further discussion of peer education.)

Sexual abuse and learning disabilities

As I outlined in the previous chapter, it was during the 1970s that awareness grew regarding the extent and nature of the sexual violence experienced by many women and children. However, it is only since the late 1980s and early

1990s (somewhat earlier in North America) that we have begun to realise what should have been apparent from the start of the process – namely, that people with learning disabilities, especially women, were not only just as likely to experience sexual abuse in the same way as other adults and children do but, moreover, that they were particularly vulnerable (Sobsey 1994). Ironically, parents of, particularly, women with learning disabilities have always known this and have been traditionally labelled as 'over-protective' by professionals for concerns which are now acknowledged to have been justified (Brown 1987).

In developing an awareness of the extent and nature of the sexual abuse, professionals have been slow to listen to what people with learning disabilities have to say about their lives. However, in recent years this has changed and the development of both sex education groups and individual work, as well as the development of more general self-advocacy networks, has enabled many people with learning disabilities to speak out about abuse they have experienced. Some teaching and resource materials available now reflect this (Brown and Stein 1997a, 1997b).

Another influential factor in the increasing awareness of abuse has been the development of HIV work outlined above – without the existence of HIV/AIDS much less would be known about the sexual abuse of people with learning disabilities. At first, the connection may not seem obvious. Despite a number of pre-existing sex education initiatives in learning disability services, which would undoubtedly have continued, it is the case that because of HIV/AIDS a number of high-profile sex education initiatives were developed for people with learning disabilities that would otherwise not have come into existence; these developments were very significant because, for the first time, they constituted a real financial commitment to the area of work and made possible the employment of specialist workers and the development of resources. It is a sad fact that it took something as negative as HIV/AIDS to release public money to be put into sexuality work with people with learning disabilities. It is also ironic that in using money set aside to try to prevent one epidemic affecting people with learning disabilities we have helped to uncover another – namely, widespread sexual abuse and exploitation.

Sexual abuse of people with learning disabilities has been defined in a variety of ways. Definitions vary in terms of both the acts and consent issues involved. A range of sexual acts are usually clustered together, including non-contact abuse – such as voyeurism and involvement in pornography –

and contact abuse – anything from sexual touch to masturbation and penetrative acts (see Brown and Turk 1992 for a review of these issues). Brown and Turk (1992) define abuse as occurring 'where sexual acts are performed on or with someone who is unwilling or unable to consent to those acts' and include within the assessment of whether an individual was able to consent both cognitive ability and inequalities of power – that is, 'whether the person had the ability to consent to sexual relationships in general and/or was able to do so without undue pressure in this particular situation' (p.49). I have previously defined it as 'any sexual contact which is unwanted and/or unenjoyed by one partner and is for the sexual gratification of the other' (McCarthy 1993, p.282).

Buchanan and Wilkins (1991) distinguish between sexual abuse as 'incest, rape, cases where violence was involved' (p.604), sexual exploitation as 'situations where a client was unable to make informed choice because of lack of knowledge about the sexual act and its consequences' (p.603) and professional abuse which they define as situations 'where the person used his/her authority to abuse the professional trust placed in him/her to gratify his/her own sexual needs' (p.604).

Matthews (1994) has made a useful contribution to the definition debate by adding that sexual abuse of a person with learning disabilities can take place 'where that person's apparent willingness is unacceptably exploited' (p.25), strengthening the argument of there being 'barriers' to consent within certain relationships (Brown and Turk 1992; Sgroi 1989). This is helpful because it moves beyond the, albeit crucial, issue of consent and indicates that although a person with learning disabilities may have understood and been willing to engage in sexual contact, they may still have been abused because of the position or motivation of the other person. Other work (McCarthy and Thompson 1997) has taken this a step further and tried to distinguish between abuse as defined by the law – for example, involving a person with a severe learning disability, staff abusing a client or someone overpowering the person using physical violence – and abuse as defined by inequality in a relationship, significant difference in ability levels or where one person's sexual needs are met at the expense of the other's. This second category of abuse, which is much less tangible and more subjective than the straightforward legal definitions, was thought to be important to investigate as clinical experience suggests that much abuse of people with learning disabilities, especially women, falls into this group (Chenoweth 1992; Crossmaker 1991; McCarthy and Thompson 1992).

As with all commentaries on sexual abuse, this one must recognise that knowledge of the true picture of sexual abuse of people with learning disabilities is inevitably incomplete. What really happens in terms of what, where, who, how and why cannot be completely known because sexual abuse, by its very nature, is a secretive and hidden activity. On top of this is the shame and guilt that both victims and perpetrators may experience, which inhibits them from speaking out about their experiences. What is known from mainstream research on sexual abuse is that most sexual abuse is never reported to the authorities (see Kelly 1988; London Rape Crisis Centre 1988). There is no reason to think that things would be any different regarding reports of sexual abuse by people with learning disabilities and, indeed, there are reasons to be more pessimistic about the proportion of abuse which is disclosed given that many people with learning disabilities have additional communication and sensory impairments.

However, the fact that we do not know everything does not mean that we do not already have a good picture of sexual abuse, as it affects people with learning disabilities, from a growing body of evidence. There have been several prevalence studies and a smaller number of incidence studies. Prevalence studies look at specific populations and record how many people have experienced abuse in their lifetime. Incidence studies look at the numbers of reported instances of abuse, within a given time period, across a defined population or catchment area – that is, the number of new cases.

Chamberlain *et al.* (1984) conducted a prevalence study in the USA. They carried out a retrospective study of case notes of 87 young women with learning disabilities who attended an adolescent clinic. They found a sexual abuse prevalence rate of 25 per cent. Elkins *et al.* (1986) conducted a very similar prevalence study at another specialist clinic in the USA and found a prevalence rate of 27 per cent. It is not clear from the report of their research whether they obtained their data from direct interviews with the women concerned or whether they relied on case notes. Hard and Plumb (1987) conducted a prevalence study in the USA in which they directly asked people with learning disabilities themselves about their experiences of abuse. The study looked at a whole population of people with learning disabilities – namely, those attending a day centre. A retrospective study of case records was carried out for all 95 subjects and this was followed by individual interviews with 65 of the original 95. (The 30 who were not interviewed were either non-verbal, unable to understand the questions, chose not to be interviewed or had left the service. The numbers of people who had been abused amongst this group is unknown but in all likelihood there would have been some.) Prevalence rates of 83 per cent for women and 32 per cent for men were reported. Also in the USA, Stromsness (1993) conducted a small prevalence study of some 27 adults with mild learning disabilities in community settings. She found a prevalence rate of 79 per cent for women and 54 per cent for men.

The first British prevalence study was carried out by Buchanan and Wilkins in 1991. They surveyed a small group of staff (total of 37) who reported knowledge of 67 cases of sexual abuse among the population of 847 people with learning disabilities they worked with – a prevalence rate of 8 per cent.

The largest and most recent British prevalence study was carried out by a colleague and myself (McCarthy and Thompson 1997). We conducted a study looking at all the 185 people with learning disabilities who had been referred to us for sex education over a five-year period. We found a prevalence rate of 61 per cent for women and 25 per cent for men.

Dunne and Power (1990) carried out a small incidence study in Ireland, looking at the 13 cases of confirmed sexual abuse that had been brought to the attention of a community learning disability team over a three-year period at a particular service (serving a total population of 1500). The data were collected from staff only and gave an incidence rate of 2.88 per thousand per annum.

The largest and most influential of the British studies are Brown et al.'s incidence studies (1992, 1995). They surveyed statutory learning disability services in the S.E. Thames Region through written questionnaires to senior managers within Health and Social Services. The resultant incidence rate in 1992 was 0.5 per cent per thousand per annum. This works out at approximately 940 cases in the UK, although this figure was revised upwards as a result of the second survey (Brown, Stein and Turk 1995), which demonstrated that services 'forgot' cases over a two-year period. These incidence figures are readily acknowledged to be 'the tip of the iceberg' and the researchers made a conscious decision to tap into knowledge at the top of the organisations which were about to take on the major commissioning role within the new internal market structures rather than closer to the service user. This decision was made on the basis that service planning decisions would be made at this level and that the capacity of services to monitor the incidence of abuse seriously was an important first step in the process of identifying need and delivering proactive services. Also, because recognition of the significance of sexual abuse for this client group has been slow to come from professional and lay audiences, it was thought important to produce the most conservative estimates and least contestable figures.

Information from other research and practice reports does indeed confirm that these figures are an underestimate. Although not a research study as such, figures released by RESPOND (a London organisation providing outreach work and sexual abuse counselling to people with learning disabilities) showed that 49 per cent of their 100 clients had been sexually abused (quoted in Marchant 1993a). These were often more able people living with minimal support from formal services but still very much at risk within the wider community. Barry (1994) also collated reports of sexual crime involving adults with learning disabilities made to the police in Kent, which suggest higher figures and indicate that there is a pool of people with learning disabilities who report directly to the police rather than through social or health care agencies.

It is apparent from these studies that both the prevalence and incidence rates vary widely. The reason for these variations is due in part to the differences in definitions of abuse, the different populations sampled and, crucially, to differences in research methods, including whether abuse rates for women and men are calculated separately or together. As has already been explained, reported instances of sexual abuse decrease the further away from the individuals the focus of the study is. Therefore, the highest rates of sexual abuse are reported when the individuals themselves are questioned (e.g. Hard and Plumb (1986); McCarthy and Thompson (1997)). When staff are questioned they can only report those cases which they know about and which they believe were true. As there are high levels of disbelief when people with learning disabilities disclose sexual abuse, it is not surprising that these figures are much lower. When senior managers are questioned they are likely only to report those instances of abuse which were formally recognised and responded to, producing yet again a much smaller number of cases (Brown and Turk 1992). (See Brown 1994 for further discussion of these issues.)

Clearly, if we want to get the most accurate picture and avoid the filtering out that takes place, there is a strong case for more research asking people with learning disabilities themselves what their experiences have been, which is precisely what I did for the research reported in this book. This approach is not without its problems, however, and these are explored in Chapter Three on methodology. Specifically in relation to researching sexual abuse, the major drawbacks are, first, that such research can only record the abusive experiences of those people with learning disabilities who have sufficient communication skills to impart the information and, second, it would be abusive in itself for researchers to descend upon people with learning disabilities, ask them questions about the most intimate and painful experiences in their lives, record the information and walk away. If people with learning disabilities are to be questioned in this way, it should be done within a meaningful and useful context for them. The need for sensitivity and trust to be built up in the research relationship is essential and, ideally, the sessions should offer people with learning disabilities something in return. This approach to research means moving away from seeing people with learning disabilities as research subjects and sources of information. For example, the data for the McCarthy and Thompson prevalence study (1997) were gained during individual sex education/counselling sessions where the sole aim *at the time of the direct contact with the client* was to provide them with a service which would benefit them.

Although estimates of incidence and prevalence rates have been made using very different methodologies, clear patterns still emerge which paint a picture of the sexual abuse of adults with learning disabilities which has similar characteristics to the sexual abuse both of adult women and of children (see, for example, Brown and Turk 1992; McCarthy and Thompson 1997). Perpetrators are overwhelmingly men, they are usually known rather than strangers, often in positions of trust and authority and have often abused before and, it is assumed (based on extrapolations from known multiple abusers), will go on to abuse other adults with learning disabilities through their connections with services. Perpetrators come from four main groups: present or past service users with learning disabilities; family members; staff and volunteers; trusted adults within the community such as family friends, neighbours, tradesmen and so on.

Both women and men are victims of sexual abuse, with studies varying in their reported figures from about 75 per cent women to almost equal numbers of men and women (see Brown, Stein and Turk 1995). Whilst a number of studies do not investigate any differences in the abuse experiences of men and women (a mistake in my view), those that do find gender differences – specifically, that women are abused more than men and that they are less likely to be believed (Hard and Plumb 1987; McCarthy and Thompson 1997). This last point is of particular significance because all available evidence suggests that most victims disclose the abuse themselves (although they are not always consciously disclosing abuse, sometimes they inadvertently reveal it). What is significant is that in most cases it is not discovered on their behalf or picked up from their behaviour or distress.

Service responses to sexual abuse

Inevitably, services have responded at different speeds and with different levels of commitment. However, the major strands of the response have tended to be the same and have been directed towards raising awareness of staff through the development of sexual abuse policies and through staff training. As indicated earlier, many local authorities, health authorities and voluntary organisations produced general sexuality and personal relationships policies during the 1980s. During the 1990s some authorities extended this work by developing policies particularly focused on abuse. The majority of these have taken one of two formats: either tackling the whole range of abuse that could be perpetrated against adults with learning disabilities or, sometimes, *all* other vulnerable adults (see, for example, Greenwich Social Services/Greenwich Health Authority undated) or more specifically looking at the sexual abuse of adults with learning disabilities (see, for example, Horizon NHS Trust 1994). Whatever the format, the function of the policies is essentially the same: to help staff and managers recognise when abuse might be happening and to guide them in correct reporting and investigating procedures. Guidance will also usually be given on ways of providing support to those people with learning disabilities who have been recently abused. What is often missing from policies is adequate guidance on, and information about, services for adult survivors of child sexual abuse and for perpetrators of sexual abuse. For those services without their own policies and strategies, *It Can Never Happen Here* (ARC/NAPSAC 1993) and *There Are No Easy Answers* (Churchill *et al.* 1997) are comprehensive documents sponsored by the Social Services Inspectorate. These were produced to guide services nation-wide on responding to the sexual abuse of and by people with learning disabilities.

Staff training initiatives specifically on the sexual abuse of people with learning disabilities have also developed during the late 1980s and 1990s. To some extent this has taken place within services by their 'in-house' training departments but also it has been conducted through the consultancy services offered by specialists in the field, myself included. In order to facilitate learning disability services in developing their staff training skills, training manuals on the subject have been produced (see Brown and Craft 1992; McCarthy and Thompson 1994b). Efforts are also being made to make sure that some mainstream sexual abuse counselling services are also made accessible to people with learning disabilities (Simpson 1994). However, as not all people with learning disabilities who have been abused would want, need or, indeed, be able to make use of long-term therapy, it is important to recognise the value of other ways of supporting people through, and after, such experiences. Valuable sex education or assertiveness groups are held in many services for people with learning disabilities. The value of women's and men's groups, and, indeed, of one-to-one advice and support sessions, is increasingly being recognised (Craft 1992; McCarthy and Thompson 1992).

The law and sexual abuse

For many years it has been acknowledged that the law often fails people with learning disabilities. This happens in many ways. There may be an absence of legislation – for example, unlike the child protection legislation, there is no law to enable statutory services to remove vulnerable adults with learning disabilities from an abusive situation in their family home unless the individuals themselves make a complaint and wish to leave. This was reviewed by the Law Commission (1995) in relation to all vulnerable adults, who recommended that 'temporary protection orders' could be used to remove a vulnerable adult to 'protective accommodation'. However, these recommendations have yet to be acted upon.

There are a number of distinct problems with the law and how it is applied in cases involving adults with learning disabilities. Laws designed to relate to adults without learning disabilities may be applied to adults with learning disabilities without any consideration given to their limited capabilities and pressures that they may have faced. This is particularly so in cases of rape or sexual abuse, which often stand or fall on the issue of consent. Consent will often be interpreted very simplistically and no account taken of why a person with learning disabilities may have consented. This also applies to many other victims of sexual crimes but is particularly poignant for people with learning disabilities. (See Chapter Five for further discussion on this issue.)

Laws may be in place and have the potential to work for the benefit of people with learning disabilities yet the way the law is applied may prevent justice from being done. There are many examples of both the police and the Crown Prosecution Service (CPS) deciding not to pursue an investigation where the victim has a learning disability. This is usually on the grounds that people with learning disabilities are thought not to make 'good enough' witnesses. Whilst it is the case that some individuals with learning disabilities do have poor memories and can only manage a disjointed and confused account of the incident(s) in question, the same could also be said of many people who do not have learning disabilities. Often, it is simply assumed that having a learning disability *per se* makes someone a poor or 'incompetent' witness.

The lack of response from the criminal justice system can be exacerbated when both the victim and the perpetrator have learning disabilities as the assumption is made that neither party will be able to give a reliable account of what happened. Hence very few perpetrators with learning disabilities are ever prosecuted (Brown, Hunt and Stein 1995; Thompson 1997).

However, caution must be exercised when alleged perpetrators with learning disabilities are apprehended by the law. Research suggests that when people with learning disabilities are arrested and the criminal justice system works towards prosecuting them, they may be disadvantaged in comparison to others. They may not always have an 'appropriate adult' to accompany them during questioning (Clare and Gudjonsson 1991), even though the codes of practice for Police and Criminal Evidence Act 1984 stipulate this. In addition, they may have a poor understanding of the caution (Gudjonsson *et al.* 1992). Appropriate responses to perpetrators with learning disabilities are discussed more fully in Chapter Six.

A recent report of research findings into crime against people with learning disabilities served to highlight their vulnerability and how infrequently justice is done (Williams 1995). But steps are now being taken to improve the situation. The work of the charitable organisation VOICE involves campaigning to make changes in the way the law itself and the legal processes affect people with learning disabilities. For example, they have successfully campaigned for relatively simple, but very effective, measures like the removal of wigs and gowns from the judges and lawyers (Hepstinall 1994). VOICE has also been awarded a Home Office grant to produce a pre-court witness pack for people with learning disabilities (Cohen 1994). Both these initiatives seek to make the court a less intimidating place for vulnerable witnesses. Indeed, work has also been undertaken at a national and strategic level on ways to make the criminal justice system more responsive to the needs of victims and witnesses who have learning disabilities (Home Office 1998).

As well as suggestions aimed to improve the criminal justice system work for people with learning disabilities, there are also suggestions about making better use of the civil law and these are discussed in Chapter Six.

Whilst it is clear that there has been much progress by both statutory and voluntary service providers and researchers over the past few years, it is important to stress that much of the knowledge about abuse and most of the thinking that has taken place on matters of prevention and responding after the event has not been informed directly by people with learning disabilities themselves. However, as I indicated earlier, this is changing and it is important to acknowledge that some people with learning disabilities are publicly speaking out about abuse. Some are not only prepared to say what has happened to them but also by sharing their feelings of injustice and anger, they have inspired other people with learning disabilities to do the same. A good example of this is the work done by a group of women with learning disabilities in Walsall. After having met privately as a women's group for some time, they decided that they wanted to share their experiences and give advice to other women who may have been abused or who feel vulnerable in their personal and social lives. The result is a video and information pack by, and for, women with learning disabilities (Walsall Women's Group 1994). The self-advocacy organisation *People First* has also provided spokespeople to appear on television programmes and at conferences to speak from the service user perspective about sexual abuse. They also provide staff training on this and related issues.

The most significant user-led development has been by a group of women with learning disabilities in East London. With support from women without learning disabilities they have campaigned, raised funds for, and designed a refuge specifically for women with learning disabilities, which is believed to be the first of its kind in the world. They named it Beverley Lewis House after a woman with learning disabilities who died of neglect. This service provides a safe place for women with learning disabilities who need to escape from any abusive situation (Powerhouse 1996a, 1996b).

The quality of the work produced by people with learning disabilities, combined with their unique perspective on the issue, indicates that researchers and service providers need to work closely with them to develop the best possible means of protecting service users from abuse and of ensuring a sensitive and consistent response to it when it does occur.

Alongside the work on the sexual abuse *against* people with learning disabilities, work has also developed (although starting later and at a slower pace) on understanding and responding to the sexual abuse *by* people with learning disabilities. Thompson (1997) has produced a very thorough examination of these issues. The most striking feature arising from this work is that all clinical, anecdotal and research evidence points to the fact that learning disabled perpetrators of sexual abuse are almost all male. Indeed, it is practically impossible to find examples in the literature of women with learning disabilities who force themselves sexually on others. As Thompson (1997) explains, there is 'substantial qualitative as well as quantitative difference' in what can be observed regarding abusive or unacceptable sexual behaviour between men and women with learning disabilities, with the isolated examples of women referring to incidents of 'flirting and clinging' to men (Sgroi 1989) and to public undressing (Mitchell 1987). More serious incidents *are* recorded (McCarthy and Thompson 1997) but these are significant in the literature only because of their rarity.

It is apparent from reviewing this literature that there is little agreement as to why men with learning disabilities sexually abuse others (and the question as to why women with learning disabilities generally do not is almost entirely ignored). There is also no consensus as to what an appropriate legal and agency response should be, although the more recent literature now offers very thorough guidance on this (Thompson and Brown 1998; Churchill *et al.* 1997). It has been suggested that whilst it is important to keep individuals and their experiences in mind at all times, it is important to understand that the abuse perpetrated by men with learning disabilities is part of a wider social phenomenon. Doing so helps services to recognise that there is much they can do to design abuse into and out of their services, such as give greater consideration to the combinations of people with very different needs who are placed together or develop women-only services (McCarthy and Thompson 1996). (See Chapter Six for a fuller discussion of these issues.)

Conclusion

As this chapter illustrates, much of what is known about the sexuality and sexual abuse of people with learning disabilities has not come directly from them. The voices of individuals describing their own experiences, and their associated thoughts and feelings, are largely missing. Also, much of the literature, certainly from the 1970s but also from the 1980s and 1990s, overlooks the fact that much of the sexual contact that takes place amongst people with learning disabilities, just as for any other people, is highly gendered in its nature. The findings of my research, presented in this book, seek to provide some of these missing perspectives.

for granted 'the ethnographer must draw the generalisations for himself, must formulate the abstract statement without the direct help of a native informant' (p.396). To make an acceptable inference the ethnographic researcher must explain why that inference is better than any other and tie in that inference with the broader knowledge of the society. Further, the inference must be able to clarify subsequent situations.

The research study in this book is based on ethnographic principles and practices. My aim was to describe and analyse the sexual lives of women with learning disabilities. My material was gained by spending time with the women, listening and asking questions. I also interpreted and drew inferences from their directly reported information, placing this in the context of observations that I made of their environments and information that came to me informally via a number of channels. Ethnographic studies are always qualitative ones, usually with a small sample size. This results in an emphasis on the depth, intensity and richness of the material obtained, rather than on providing a sweeping overview. The findings presented in the next chapter clearly fit into that pattern. Likewise, as with a lot of other ethnographic studies, it is in the tradition of what Fielding (1993) calls 'pathbreaking' research – that is, exploring the hitherto unknown or obscure; this research offers the first *in-depth* insight into the way women with learning disabilities experience their sexual lives.

Ethnographic researchers have tended to emphasise that it is important for researchers to learn how to understand and speak the same language as their subjects. With its roots in anthropology, this would have meant, in many cases, actually learning a foreign language. But even when the researcher and researched share the same native language it is important not to assume that each knows what the other is talking about. Some of the difficulties of interviewing people with learning disabilities are discussed later but, for me, it was also important to be aware that many people with learning disabilities (particularly those living in hospitals) have slang terms or jargon just like any other sub-culture. For example, being 'up the pole' means getting angry or losing your temper, and not, as some might assume, a slang term for being pregnant. Clearly, in the context of my research, it was very important to know that!

This research differs from some other ethnographic studies in that there is no element of participant observation. With regards to the women's general life experiences, there was no possibility of my living alongside the women with learning disabilities in their 'natural' settings. Therefore, I could not gain first-hand experience of what their daily lives were like. I do have insights into this from having worked in a variety of institutional and community-based learning disability services for a considerable period of time but I am the first to admit that this is not the same.

With regards to the women's sexual experiences, which, after all, form the *raison d'être* of this research, these are also not amenable to direct study. Because in society people's actual sexual activity (as opposed to representations of it) is considered an essentially private matter between the people concerned, the only ethically acceptable way of directly observing people's sexual behaviour is if the subjects volunteer freely to take part. As my research subjects were not volunteers, and, moreover, because people with learning disabilities are generally considered to be more easily suggestible than the general population, it would have been completely unethical even to suggest direct observation. Added to this, the researcher's feelings and needs have to be taken into account and I certainly had no wish to do direct observations. Therefore, I was entirely dependent on the women's first-hand accounts. Whilst this may be a departure from traditional ethnographic studies, it is a method consistent with most other, usually much larger scale, research projects into sexual behaviour (e.g. Kinsey 1948, 1953; Hite 1976, 1981). However, direct observations have been undertaken by other sex researchers (e.g. Masters and Johnson).

A political perspective on disability research

The oppression of people with disabilities can be seen on a number of levels. For example, discrimination against people with disabilities can be measured by their lack of equal access to employment (Labour Research 1992; Ravaud, Madiot and Ville 1992), housing (Dunn 1990; Fielding 1990), health care (Bax, Smyth and Thomas 1988) and by almost any other factor one cares to mention. As a result of such discrimination, people with disabilities (like women, Black people, gay men and lesbians) have formed social and political movements to fight their oppression and campaign for equality. It is in this context that in recent years a small number of writers and researchers, who often themselves have physical disabilities (and some of whom are also feminists), have started to challenge many aspects of research on disabled people. Their challenges revolve around the lack of research in the first place, how that research which has been done has not proved itself useful to disabled people's lives, how it has been done on disabled people by non-disabled people and how it has pathologised individual disabled people and their problems (Oliver 1990, 1992). In short, 'disability research has, in the main, been part of the problem rather than part of the solution' (Morris 1992, p.157).

Oliver (1990) states that: 'the process of the [research] interview is oppressive, reinforcing onto isolated, individual disabled people the idea that the problems they experience in everyday living are a direct result of their own personal inadequacies or financial limitations' (p.8).

That being the case, positive and practical suggestions are put forward by writers such as Morris and Oliver which are very useful – that is, to contextualise research within a disability rights perspective, which identifies that it is the non-disabled world which denies opportunities to, and oppresses, disabled people. Furthermore, some disabled people are demanding the right to be given the means (including access to education, jobs and resources) to do research themselves. In the absence of this they demand to be consulted about the type of research done, its methods and the use to which it will be put. It is suggested that the methodology of research must change and be built upon trust and respect, building in participation and reciprocation, so that research itself would become part of a developmental process which includes education and political action (Oliver 1992).

The political perspective taken on disability research referred to above is written by people with, and/or focuses on, physical disability and assumes that the subjects of the research would have the intellectual capacity to contribute to the research process in the ways described above. More recently, however, a separate, and small, body of literature has developed which is written almost exclusively by non-disabled researchers about working collaboratively with people with learning disabilities (Minkes *et al.* 1995; Townsley 1995; Young 1996). This literature points out that, unlike in the physical disability field, the pressure to make the research process accessible to those who traditionally had been only research subjects has not come from people with learning disabilities themselves. Nevertheless, the literature suggests that it is both possible and desirable to involve people with learning disabilities at all stages of the process, from setting the research agenda to disseminating the results. However, whilst it may be possible, it is rarely done and those who have made efforts in this direction do admit to particular difficulties with certain parts of research. For example, Minkes *et al.* (1995) point out that including people with learning disabilities in 'arguably the most complex part of the research process' (p.97) – that is, data analysis, has proved particularly problematic, whilst Swain *et al.* (1998) refer to the 'cosmetic' involvement of people with learning disabilities in presenting research findings, especially in academic papers.

Whilst I agree that involving people with learning disabilities in research, as researchers, is a development in the right direction (see p.106), I also feel that those who are proposing such moves need to give more consideration to the different contexts in which research happens in learning disability services. When work is commissioned by a service and/or is funded by a government department or major funding body (Minkes *et al.* 1995), it may well be possible for all concerned to invest their time and financial resources in making the research process accessible to people with learning disabilities. However, not all research is conducted under these conditions. Practice-based research, such as mine, is often done in rather different circumstances (McCarthy 1995). Throughout the whole of the study reported here only the actual time spent interviewing women with learning disabilities was done during my work time. Everything else has been done in my own time. In addition, there was no funding for the research other than my employer paying approximately half of my tuition fees to the university and my travel expenses. Other researchers, with little or no funding and very limited work time available, would find themselves in a very similar position to mine – that is, effectively not in a position to provide resources or support for any people with learning disabilities with the means to do the research themselves, or even to work alongside us.

In addition to this is that fact that the social model of disability (an analysis of disability as a function of material, economic, social and cultural barriers) has not been so rigorously explored in relation to people with learning, as opposed to physical, disabilities (Stalker 1998). In relation to research, Walmsley (1994) has offered a critique of whether and to what extent it is realistic or helpful to imagine people with learning disabilities taking control over the research process. Few other researchers and writers have engaged with Walmsley's arguments however – possibly because publicly acknowledging or accepting that having an intellectual impairment may effectively exclude people from certain pursuits (research, after all, is an intellectual exercise first and foremost) is deemed to be politically incorrect.

In my study I certainly informed the women with learning disabilities whom I interviewed what I was doing in very simple terms – for example, 'I am talking to women about sex, so I can learn more about it and try to make sure women get the help they need'. The actual words 'research', 'methods', 'policy', etc, would not necessarily have been used because they were not familiar terms to most of the people I worked with. But, nevertheless, I tried to see that the women had a basic understanding of what I was doing. However, this was to try to gain their informed consent (for a fuller discussion on this see p.104) and it was not a consultation process. Although each individual woman had to agree to my asking her questions, she was not asked whether she agreed with the whole tenet of the research in the first place. That said, some women did spontaneously say that they thought it was a good idea and if any had said it was a bad idea and why, I would certainly have listened carefully to that.

Minkes *et al.* (1995) suggest that where it is not possible to involve people with learning disabilities as researchers, all research needs to focus on their needs and ensure that they are enabled to express their opinions and interests. Morris (1992) suggests two main ground rules that non-disabled researchers should follow. The first is to turn the spotlight on the oppressors rather than the oppressed and the second is to put the personal experiences of individual disabled people into a social and political context whilst, at the same time, giving a voice to the 'absent' research subject. These were certainly my intentions in this research study.

Morris also asserts that it is not very helpful to talk about disabled women experiencing a double disadvantage because the negative images of disadvantage can contribute to the actual experience of oppression. I agree that this is the case but, at the same time, believe that it is surely not very helpful to avoid stating an obvious truth: that living as a disabled person in a world that highly values a lack of disability and living as a woman in a patriarchal society *is* to experience a double disadvantage (Deegan and Brooks 1985; Hutchinson *et al.* 1993; Williams 1992). Similarly, to be a Black woman in a society which discriminates against both Black people and women or to be a lesbian in a society which discriminates against same-sex relationships and against women is to experience double disadvantage. Indeed, some Black disabled women have spoken about their experience of 'triple discrimination' (Francis 1996). Clearly, these are very complex issues for the experience of being disabled or Black or a woman is different for individual people, even though they share some of the same characteristics. People's own personal resources, such as their family and cultural background, their own personality and their material resources, will inter-relate with factors of external oppression to produce different sets of circumstances and different feelings of oppression associated with them. Nevertheless, it seems unhelpful to avoid all reference to 'double disadvantage' for in doing so an opportunity is lost to highlight the fact that there are many layers of oppression in operation. As long as it is made clear by the commentator that s/he believes there is nothing wrong with any of the above states of being *per se*, but rather that it is the responses that these 'conditions' generate in people (who, usually, do not share them) which are at fault, then I am fairly comfortable with the phrase and concept of 'double disadvantage' and at times in this research I highlight where I think it is operating for women with learning disabilities (see p.214).

Feminist research methodology

Feminist research grew out of the second wave of feminism in the United States and Western Europe from the 1970s onwards. As women were analysing the impact of gender power relations in all spheres of life, it was inevitable that traditional research methodology would be scrutinised and found to be as male dominated as any other academic pursuit at that time. Research methodology was, therefore, reconstructed by feminists to reflect the changing gender politics and gender relations of wider society.

There now seems to be a general consensus of opinion in the literature that there are no such things as feminist research methods (i.e. techniques, specific sets of research practice). Claims that had been made in the late 1970s/early 1980s regarding the divide between quantitative research methods being essentially male, and, therefore, bad for women, versus qualitative research methods being essentially female, and, therefore, good, have largely faded away (Stanley and Wise 1993). Conversely, there is a consensus that there is such a thing as feminist methodology (i.e. a framework or perspective, a set of guiding principles). These principles concern the research process itself – that is, who is researching whom, what about, how and why – as well as broader issues – such as the use to which the research may be put.

With regard to the research process, the need for reflexivity has been emphasised by many feminist researchers (see, for example, Acker, Barry and Esseveld 1983; Clegg 1985; Harding 1987; Stanley 1990). Reflexivity is a reaction to the claims of objectivity that had traditionally formed part of the positivist research paradigm and which was based on a belief that the social world could be studied in the same way as the natural world. Reflexivity is based on a belief that knowledge obtained from research is dependent on the assumptions underpinning it and the methods used to obtain it. Consequently, both the researcher's assumptions and her/his methods must be made explicit. Some writers go further and assert that biographical details such as the researcher's class, race, culture, gender, beliefs and behaviours should be 'placed in the same critical plane as the overt subject matter, thereby recovering the entire research process for scrutiny in the results of research' (Harding 1987, p.9). However, as explained above with reference to the politics of disability research, such biographical details do not necessarily tell you anything very much about individual people. Nevertheless, at different points in this research study (where it has seemed relevant) I have attempted to 'place' myself, both as an individual and in relation to my research subjects. This is usually in terms of explaining shared experiences rather than biographical facts. Moreover, considerable space has been given to reflecting on the actual research methods used (see below).

Another central principle of feminist methodology is the rejection of a traditional androcentric bias, which subsumes women's experiences into men's – that is, assumes that women's experiences will be the same as men's and therefore uses generic terms to describe research subjects and their actions. This is certainly true with regard to people with learning disabilities, who, in the professional literature and/or services provided for them, are usually referred to as *people* with learning disabilities and not as women and men, or as girls and boys, with different and potentially conflicting needs and experiences (Atkinson and Walmsley 1995). By choosing to focus this research study on the sexual experiences of women with learning disabilities, I was actively seeking to redress some of the traditional androcentrism.

Also fundamental to feminist methodology is a rejection of the traditional public/private split (see p.36), an ideology which has placed men's concerns and activities in the public, therefore noteworthy, sphere of life and women's concerns and activities in the private, therefore unimportant, sphere of life. Feminist research methodology takes from feminist activism the belief that the 'personal is political'. 'To see the personal as political means to see the private as public' (MacKinnon 1987, p.148). Thus women's experiences and men's behaviour (as so much of the former is dependent on the latter) are forced onto the agenda for public scrutiny. Much of this research study (especially that which relates to sexual abuse) involves placing the private experiences of women with learning disabilities in a public and political context. This research study follows the path laid down by activists in the women's movement as well as by other feminist researchers, without which the exposure of the extent of sexual abuse of women and children by men would not have been possible. Sadly, as a society we are nowhere near a complete picture of the true extent and nature of abuse, but hopefully this study will be a useful contribution to the wider picture.

Moving away from the research process to the purpose and outcomes of research, there is agreement amongst feminist methodologists that research must aim to be of use to women in the sense that it contributes to challenging and ending oppression (Stanley and Wise 1993). Just as some ethnographers (e.g. Spradley 1979) have argued that knowledge for its own sake is not a good enough reason to undertake what might be intrusive, lengthy and costly research, so feminist researchers have also emphasised that 'the questions an oppressed group want answered are rarely requests for so-called pure truth. Instead, they are queries about how to change its conditions' (Harding 1987, p.8).

Because in certain contexts knowledge can give access to power and because research findings can be distorted and used for purposes other than those which were intended, the feminist researcher has a responsibility to see that the research is, at the very least, intended to benefit women's interests and do what she can to prevent it from being 'misused'. In relation to this, Finch (1984) describes how her fears that her research findings would be misinterpreted and used against the women she had interviewed about their children's playgroups prevented her from writing them up for some considerable time. I share these concerns in relation to my work on sexuality and learning disability and have publicly expressed concerns about other people misusing my findings:

> Those who work and write about the sexuality of people with learning disabilities are acutely aware that we do so against a background of oppression towards them. Their historical institutionalisation and segregation was due to complex reasons, but issues of sexuality were central to this process. Ideas about the supposedly uncontrolled nature of their sexuality sat side by side with ideas about their sexual vulnerability in society. There is a danger in that in highlighting the vulnerability of many women with learning disabilities to sexual abuse and the extent of the sexual abuse that is perpetrated by men with learning disabilities, that these factors will be used by some people to try to prove that what are now rightly considered as old fashioned and inherently damaging ideas were right after all. There is also the risk that such work will be used by to strengthen some of the more general essentialist ideas about women's sexual passivity and men's sexual aggression. I am the last person to want to turn the clock back this way and I am concerned about being accused

> of perpetuating stereotypes. Yet at the same time I do not want to be
> pressured into keeping quiet, as I believe it does a great disservice to
> women with learning disabilities in particular. I am hoping to find a
> space within the learning disability field and within feminism where we
> can acknowledge what is happening and find ways of changing it.
> (McCarthy 1996a, p.127)

Despite concerns that what one makes public may be reinterpreted and,
indeed, misinterpreted by others, most researchers, myself included, do make
the decision to publish our work. Whose interests we serve by doing so is
open to question but it is an example both of the power we have as researchers over those we research as well as a way of coping with one of the demands
of an academic career.

The question as to who can research whom is central to all three research
perspectives I have discussed in this chapter. Research is still largely carried
out by those who have power on those who have little or no power. This is
clear from a disability research perspective, where able-bodied people have
invited themselves into the lives of disabled people, asking all manner of
questions and, in the case of medical research, carrying out all kinds of
intrusive and abusive procedures without regard for the feelings of the
individuals on the receiving end (Morris 1992). It is also the case that
non-disabled researchers have traditionally paid little attention to the fact
that they can very easily (sometimes inadvertently, sometimes deliberately)
use their advantage in intellect and status to get people with learning
disabilities to speak freely about otherwise private and protected topics of
discussion (Swain, Heyman and Gillman 1998; Thompson 1998).

Within the traditions of sociology, it has long been recognised that the
most powerful – that is, white, middle-class, able-bodied – heterosexual men
have protected themselves from scrutiny (Park 1978) and this has produced
what Liazos (1972) describes as a sociology of 'nuts, sluts and perverts'. It is,
therefore, incumbent upon feminists, amongst others, not always to 'study
down' but also to 'study up' and 'study along' and study ourselves. Whilst
efforts have certainly been made in that direction, feminist research cannot
really claim to be egalitarian for it is still largely 'us' (what Stanley and Wise
(1993) call the 'theorizing researching elite' of feminists) researching 'them'
– that is, women. I cannot make any other claims for this research. However, I
think it is important to note that despite the fact that this research fits
theoretically into the oppressive model of one of the elite 'us' researching
'them', this is not necessarily how it feels to the subjects of the research. First,

this is because the women with learning disabilities I interviewed did not appear to have any awareness or understanding that there are such people as academics or feminists. Second, on a more general level, my knowledge of, and skills in, interviewing, combined with my natural inclination and conscious efforts to be pleasant, friendly and respectful of the women's dignity and privacy, led to a situation whereby the women seemed to feel valued rather than oppressed by me. Having lengthy, one-to-one conversations on a regular basis with someone who is treating them with respect is, sadly, a luxury afforded to all too few people with learning disabilities. It is, therefore, valued when it does occur, regardless of the wider context.

Within the field of ethnography it has been claimed that some groups are especially vulnerable and have a right not to be researched (Fielding 1993). No examples were given nor was the point elaborated, but one could speculate that individuals or groups who do not understand the nature of the research might come into that category. Furthermore, using 'captive groups' (again, no examples were given) for research has been described as 'anti-feminist' (Ehrlich 1976 cited in Stanley and Wise 1993, p.37). I do not agree with either of the above statements for to agree with them would mean that no research could ever be done on children, adults with severe learning disabilities, anybody in prisons, hospitals, schools or other institutions. To a large extent, people's vulnerability can be protected by the use of anonymity and confidentiality and by the researcher being sensitive to people's dignity and rights of privacy. Not to research people because they are perceived to be generally vulnerable and/or because they are (perhaps literally) a captive group means they could be rendered even more vulnerable as there will be an ignorance about their circumstances and how they are treated. However, balancing the right or need of the public to know about individuals' experiences and the right and ability of those individuals to protect themselves from intrusion and public scrutiny is rarely acknowledged in the research literature (see Swain, Heyman and Gillman 1998 for a notable exception).

To summarise thus far, for this study I chose in-depth qualitative research methods which fit into both the academic traditions of ethnography and feminist research principles whilst, at the same time, meeting some of the set criteria of good disability research principles – that is, giving people with disabilities an opportunity to voice their experiences and opinions. The research methodology fits into the ethnographic tradition because I sought to understand and describe the experiences of one set of people to another. It is from a disability rights perspective because it actively challenges the pathologising of individual people with disabilities and firmly sets their experiences in a wider social context. My methodology was simultaneously from a feminist perspective because it focused on women's experiences, seeing these in both personal and political contexts; it also challenges women's oppression and its aim was to improve the lives of women with learning disabilities.

Particular considerations for researching sensitive topics

There is a small but growing body of literature concerned with the process and practicalities of researching sensitive topics (see Lee 1993; Renzetti and Lee 1993). In relation to research, the label 'sensitive' is sometimes not defined at all and a common-sense approach is taken as if the term were self-explanatory (Renzetti and Lee 1993). Common-sense definitions are useful in so far as most people would understand them to include topics which are difficult or taboo to talk about socially, such as sex or death (Farberow 1963). However, such self-explanatory definitions are not useful in understanding research where the *topic* itself may not be particularly sensitive but the *context* of the research is, such as Brewer's (1990) research on routine policing in Northern Ireland.

'Sensitive' meaning 'socially sensitive' research has been defined as being more or less synonymous with 'controversial' – Sieber and Stanley (1988) define it as 'studies in which there are potential consequences or implications, either directly for the participants in the research or for the class of individuals represented by the research' (p.49). This is a very broad definition and, I would suggest, not very clear because it could encompass positive or negative, large or small consequences. Lee (1993) offers an alternative definition of sensitive research as being that which 'potentially poses a substantial threat to those who are or who have been involved in it' (p.4). At a first reading it is hard to see how my research study, which most people would consider to be sensitive, could be understood as posing a substantial threat to the women involved, given that anonymity has been provided. However, Lee goes on to further define 'threat' as either being an 'intrusive threat', in that it deals with areas of life which are private, stressful or sacred; as possibly revealing information which is stigmatising or incriminating in some way; or where the research impinges on political alignments – that is, it exposes the vested interests of powerful persons or institutions and/or exposes coercion and dominance. As my research clearly involved delving into a very private sphere of life, does reveal (albeit limited) information about some of the women themselves which is stigmatising (such as accepting money for sex) and does expose sexual coercion and dominance of some groups and individuals by others, then on all three counts it would be classed as sensitive.

As well as being a potential threat to the subjects of the research, it is argued that some kinds of sensitive research pose a potential threat to the researcher. Research on human sexuality is singled out as being the area most likely to lead to this, with researchers being seen, certainly in the past although less so today, as 'morally suspect' (Plummer 1975). Although it has not been my own experience, some sexuality researchers (see Troiden 1987 for a fuller discussion of this) experience 'occupational stigma' because of their study of sexuality. They feel their work is trivialised, that their professional interest in sexuality is deemed to be related to their own personal sexual failings or excesses and are assumed to share the same sexual characteristics as those they study (Fisher undated), particularly being assumed to be lesbian or gay if they study homosexuality. It is also suggested that academic promotion may be hindered, as the topic is deemed to be too specialised as well as controversial. As I have indicated, I have not experienced this 'occupational stigma' myself. This is possibly because there is a well-established strand of sexuality work within the learning disability field and, as the review of the literature in Chapter Two demonstrates, I am certainly not working in isolation. However, I have been aware that assumptions have been made about by own sexual experiences based on my professional interests. For example, it has been assumed that I must have experienced sexual abuse myself because I am 'so' interested in the sexual abuse of women with learning disabilities. This is not the case, although the assumption itself is an interesting one – it would not, after all, be assumed of a speech therapist that they had a personal history of problems with verbal communication. Also, because I have publicly (through my writing and conference presentations) been very critical of much of men's sexual behaviour and of the way heterosexual masculinity is constructed, I know it has been assumed that I must be either lesbian or celibate, when in fact I am neither.

However, this is not to suggest that if researchers do share certain characteristics with the subjects of their research, this in any way invalidates their involvement. On the contrary, a shared interest or experience can enrich a researcher's work and certainly is not necessarily a factor which leads to the research or researcher being less objective than another person. The need for reflexivity, which is outlined above with regard to feminist research methodology, would indicate a need for the researcher to explore the effects of shared experiences on their work. For my part, I assume that the assumptions made about me on the basis of my work in this field remain in the realm of the personal and have little or no discernible effect on my professional life. Certainly, to date, I have had no trouble getting my work taken seriously and although the range of my work *is* narrow and specialised, that, in so far as it is a problem, is a self-inflicted one.

It has been argued (for example, by MacIntyre 1982) that certain areas of human life are too private and too sensitive to be researched and, therefore, ought not to be: 'certain areas of personal and social life should be specially protected. Intimacy cannot exist where everything is disclosed, sanctuary cannot be sought where no place is inviolate' (p.188).

This would be all very well if everything that happens under the cloak of intimacy is positive, lawful and healthy and that sanctuary is only sought by those who have nothing to hide. However, much of feminist research and activism over many years has been devoted to exposing the exploitation of women within intimate relationships in the supposed sanctuary of their own homes. Indeed, research studies on sensitive topics are important precisely because 'they challenge taken-for-granted ways of seeing the world' (Lee 1993, p.2) and 'address some of society's most pressing social and policy issues' (Sieber and Stanley 1988, p.5).

Just as I argue against those ethnographers who felt that certain groups of people should be protected from research, I would argue against certain topics or life experiences not being open to research. It seems to me that if people are willing to share their experiences and certain conditions are in place to ensure their contributions are respected and as individuals they are not exploited, there is no subject that cannot be researched. Moreover, the arguments that certain people or certain topics should be avoided because of the potential negative effects research can have on the subjects overlooks the potential positive effects that researching sensitive topics can have. Kvale (1983 cited in McLeod 1994) argues that a well carried out research interview can be an enriching experience for the subjects. Kennedy Bergen, regarding her interviews with women who had experienced marital rape, states that most of her subjects 'claimed that speaking about their experiences was cathartic and said they were grateful to have a sympathetic listener' (1993, p.209). In addition, there is the positive desire expressed by some research participants, including those with learning disabilities (Booth and

Booth 1994) and at least one of mine in this study, to use their own painful experiences to help others.

Moving on to the particular conditions needed to safeguard the rights of subjects involved in the research of sensitive topics, it is clear that few, if any, are exclusive to this work. Rather, they are an extension or elaboration of good practice in research generally. McLeod (1994) describes a 'small set of basic ethical principles' derived from counselling and medical practice which need to be applied: 'These are *beneficence* (acting to enhance client well being), *nonmaleficence* (avoiding doing harm to the clients), *autonomy* (respecting the right of the person to take responsibility for himself or herself) and *fidelity* (treating everyone in a fair and just manner)' (1994, p.165).

Although preserving the anonymity of research subjects is not explicitly mentioned in McLeod's list (possibly because it may seem like stating the obvious), this is, of course, of the utmost importance.

It is generally accepted in the literature that whilst informed consent of subjects is important for all research studies, the more sensitive the topic, the greater the need for ascertaining truly informed consent (Renzetti and Lee 1993). McLeod (1994) goes into some detail about what informed consent actually means and why it may be difficult or impossible to obtain it from certain people – for example, children or adults in a highly distressed state. But what the sensitive research literature fails to do is to offer any clear guidelines on proceeding (or not) if informed consent cannot be obtained. The ethics of research with subjects who cannot give informed consent, because of intellectual limitations and/or lifetimes of conditioning to comply with other people's wishes, are not addressed. Rather, it is implied that problems regarding informed consent can all be overcome if handled in a sensitive enough manner. Some researchers engaged in work with people with learning disabilities, including myself, come to different conclusions and this is an issue I address in more depth below.

One of the other primary concerns in researching sensitive topics is the distress that may be experienced by the subjects during the actual interviews. It has already been stated that this is far from inevitable but, clearly, there is greater potential for distress with sensitive topics than innocuous ones. There is conflicting advice in the literature about dealing with distress – whilst all advice indicates the need to anticipate that distress may occur and plan in advance how to support subjects at the time and afterwards, thereafter researchers approach the matter differently. Brannen and Collard (1982) argue that although researchers need to be supportive and seek to contain highly emotionally charged scenes, it is essential for a researcher not to become a counsellor to the subjects; Swain, Heyman and Gillman (1998) also felt that providing counselling to research subjects was unacceptable. Kennedy Bergen (1993), on the other hand, takes the opposite approach and argues, with reference to a woman who had become particularly distressed, that 'it was not problematic for me to comfort this woman (both during and after the interview) as I had not compartmentalised my identity into counsellor, researcher and woman' (p.208).

This is the approach I adopted with the women with learning disabilities I worked with in this study, partly because it seems more intellectually and practically sound and partly because the context in which I carried out the research (i.e. during sex education/counselling sessions) effectively demanded it. Research with people with learning disabilities takes place in a variety of contexts and it is not uncommon for research data to be gathered as part of a broader involvement in people's lives, either as direct service providers, therapists or managers (Hart and Bond 1995). For me to have tried not to be a counsellor during the research part of my sessions with the women would have been particularly confusing for those women whose understanding of my research role was limited (this links with the issue of informed consent, which is addressed in more depth below). In addition, I made an ethical decision that were there ever to be a conflict of interest between my need for research material and a woman's need for support or therapeutic help, the latter would always take precedence.

Given the nature of the topics discussed during sensitive research, the demands such discussions may make on the subjects and the skills required of the researcher to conduct the interviews in a respectful way, it is clear that there is some overlap between the research and counselling elements of such a task. When the two are conflated in this way it is usual to consider what research has to offer counselling. Obviously, the knowledge gained from research, such as greater insights into people's behaviour and feelings, can contribute to the delivery of more effective counselling services. What is often overlooked, however, is what counselling and good interviewing skills have to offer research. McLeod (1994) argues convincingly that counselling theories can help to make sense of the relationship between the researcher and the subject and the effects of this relationship on what is said or not said. In addition, he claims that experienced counsellors may make good researchers in the sense that they will have skills in establishing rapport, be good listeners and ask and answer questions constructively and sensitively –

in short, they will have developed the necessary interpersonal skills to facilitate discussion on topics which are hard for most people to talk about. In my own research my prior experience not only of counselling women with learning disabilities on sexuality issues but also working with people with learning disabilities more broadly was invaluable in helping me to both design and conduct the research interviews (see below for a fuller discussion on methods).

Interviewing people with learning disabilities

As I have remarked elsewhere, 'interviewing people with learning difficulties is not a fundamentally different process from interviewing anybody else' (McCarthy 1991, p.24). The researchers still have to decide what the focus of the interview is going to be, an interview schedule has to be drawn up, respondents have to be selected, the questions put and the answers and inter-action analysed. However, having said that interviewing people with learning disabilities is not wholly different from interviewing other people, it also has to be acknowledged that it is not exactly the same. There are differ-ences, some obvious, some more hidden.

Specific considerations

One of the more obvious considerations is that the ability to answer ques-tions is in itself partly a function of intelligence (Flynn 1986) and people with learning disabilities, by definition, have an intellectual impairment. The body of literature regarding interviewing people with learning disabilities is small and within it there does appear to be agreement that the way questions are worded has more significance for people with learning disabilities than for the general population. In other words, bearing in mind the intellectual impairment, people's ability to answer accurately can be maximised or mini-mised depending on how the questions are put. One of the researchers in this field, Sigelman, along with her colleagues, has demonstrated that people with learning disabilities have a greater tendency than other people to choose the last option in either/or and multiple choice questions (sometimes referred to as *recency*). This tendency in some people with learning disabilities is well known to those who work closely with them. However, despite this tendency, Sigelman *et al.* still recommend the use of either/or questions in preference to questions requiring yes/no answers (1981a). This is because the tendency towards acquiescence (answering yes to a question regardless of its content) is even more marked with this population (1981b). The tendency to acquiesce (long since recognised also in the non-disabled population in surveys, for example Wells 1963) becomes more pronounced the greater the degree of learning disability and the more abstract and subjective the question. However, the tendencies amongst people with learning disabilities towards recency and acquiescence, whilst widely accepted, have also been subject to challenge. For example, Simons, Booth and Booth (1989) argue that asking the kind of questions Sigelman *et al.* did in 'laboratory' conditions was likely to generate uncertainty and doubt in the minds of the subjects, something they describe as 'a positive inducement to acquiesce'. More recently, Rapley and Antaki (1996) have provided a very convincing critique of Sigelman *et al.*'s work. They suggest that people with learning disabilities are not inherently prone to acquiescence. They argue that what appears to be straightforward acquiescence is, in fact, a highly complex process and can only be understood by analysing the perceptions and motivations of both interviewer and interviewee and the dynamics between them.

Even amongst those who accept that acquiescence does occur, precisely why people are more likely to answer yes to a question rather than no when they are uncertain is not often discussed. However, Gudjonsson (1986), as a result of his research, suggests that 'affirmative answers are perceived to be more acceptable to the interviewer and are consequently less likely to be challenged than "no" or "don't know" answers' (p.199). Wyngaarden (1981) suggests the use of open-ended questions to avoid the above-mentioned response biases and this certainly makes sense theoretically. However, it has been noted by other researchers, notably Booth and Booth (1994), that open-ended questions often do not facilitate people with learning disabilities in talking freely and fluently. They found, as I did with many of my interviewees, that 'generally speaking [our] informants were more inclined to answer questions with a single word, a short phrase or the odd sentence' (p.36).

It is apparent then, that either/or, yes/no and open-ended questions all have their limitations when interviewing people with learning disabilities. What happens in practice is that researchers have to find their own style, based on a likely mixture of the above approaches, and vary it accordingly for each individual. For instance, at an early stage in my interviews I 'tested' each woman's tendency to choose the last option in either/or questions. Although the need to begin interviews with an open mind and 'test' people's abilities is recognised in the literature (Booth and Booth 1994), the actual difficulty in doing this is not explicitly acknowledged. For instance, I used the technique of repeating questions and reversing the order of the options to test for the tendency for recency. But, clearly, this technique has to be used sparingly and/or done with tact and skill to avoid interviewees feeling patronised or irritated by it. That said, it is necessary to make some assessment of this kind and if I felt that any individual woman did tend to choose the last option, I would endeavour to avoid this kind of question where possible. Alternatively, if I could anticipate a likely response, I would place this as first rather than last option so the woman was forced to give the matter some thought. To give a concrete example, I expected (on the basis of all my previous work in this field and on traditional social and sexual expectations of women and men) the women to say that it was men who initiated sexual activity with them and not the other way around. Therefore, I would phrase the question 'who starts the sex, the man or you?' This meant that women who would automatically say the last option had to take a moment to think whether that was the correct answer (for her) or not.

I tended to repeat and rephrase questions often, something which is suggested in the literature as being important to 'elicit the most complete response' (Wyngaarden 1981, p.109). I also tended to repeat, reflect and summarise the women's answers back to them as we went along. This was to check both that I had understood what they had said and that they had said what they meant to say. As well as a concrete way of demonstrating respect for the women and what they were saying, this was an important step in terms of trying to empower the women. In other words, it was a way in which I tried to ensure that individually and collectively the women's own voices were heard.

As many people with learning disabilities find the concepts of time and frequency very difficult, Flynn (1986) suggests these are best avoided in interviews. Booth and Booth (1994) assert that in their research (on the parenting experiences of people with learning disabilities) these problems could be overcome if researchers were satisfied with approximations rather than accuracy and if concrete markers of time were used − such as Christmases, holidays, children's ages. Whilst these are undoubtedly helpful techniques, it must also be recognised that the subjects in the Booths' research, as parents, were at the more able end of the learning disability spectrum and, therefore, likely to have least problems with the abstract concepts of time and frequency. My experience in this research was that it was indeed problematic for most of the women to say how recently or long ago something happened and also how frequently or infrequently they experienced something. I certainly had to be satisfied with approximations and tried to develop a 'sense' based on the entirety of what a woman said and how often or long ago something may have happened. I was satisfied with this, partly because there was no other option and partly because I was trying to gain an insight into the woman's own understanding of her experience, and so the details of when and how often something may have happened were not always relevant anyway.

Rapport

The literature on the methodology of interviewing people with learning disabilities also deals with ethical issues and building rapport. Atkinson (1989) and Booth and Booth (1994) both emphasise the need to develop good rapport with interviewees with learning disabilities. In these studies subjects were interviewed in their own homes (sometimes mentioned in the general literature on interviewing as having great significance in itself as a way of establishing rapport (e.g. Kennedy Bergen 1993). Atkinson places a lot of importance on the informality of the interview, with the researcher behaving as a guest – for example, always taking a gift for the interviewee (flowers, cake, etc) and complimenting the person's house, photographs or ornaments. Booth and Booth never visited any of their interviewees carrying briefcases or clipboards and tried hard not be associated in the minds of their subjects with representatives of any statutory agencies. This was because many of their subjects, like other parents with learning disabilities, had had tense and difficult relationships with professionals involved in child protection work (Booth and Booth 1995). However, they recognised the difficulties inherent in this – as middle-class people working with predominantly working-class parents, they felt conspicuous by their accents, clothes, cars, etc.

My situation was different in that I was never seeing anyone just for research purposes. All interviews were carried out in my role as sex educator and, therefore, I was clearly identified as a worker in the service and no attempt was made to disguise or play down this fact. Most of my interviews were conducted in the office/counselling room that all other sex education sessions took place in, rather than the person's own home. Whilst this may have lent the interviews a more formal air, the reality of working in the homes of many people with learning disabilities must be recognised. All except one of my interviewees (in hospital and the community) lived in shared accommodation and in order to have a strictly private conversation often the only available place was the woman's bedroom. As the rooms were often rather small and people did not always have chairs in their bedroom, in effect this sometimes meant both researcher and interviewee having to sit on the bed to discuss sexual matters. This shifts the atmosphere from the informal to the intimate. Whilst it did not appear to be an actual problem in any of the interviews (or, indeed, in my wider counselling and educational work with women with learning disabilities), it has, nevertheless, always felt to me to be quite inappropriate and I always avoided it where possible.

Wherever the interview took place, I always made conscious efforts to create an informal atmosphere. Women were always offered tea or coffee and biscuits – this offering of refreshments is particularly important as it is a way of signifying that this is intended to be an informal and friendly experience. It distinguishes the session from other kinds of help people might receive in services (doctors, psychologists, teachers, etc. do not, to my knowledge, generally offer people cups of tea in their offices or classrooms). As a gesture, it symbolises the fact that I wish to give something to the women as well as get something from them. The fact that the offer of refreshments was never, ever refused also indicates its importance. Likewise, where I did interview women in their own homes, I always accepted the offer of a drink, even if I did not want one. It is interesting to note, however, that women did not usually offer me any refreshments unless they were prompted by support staff to do so. There is no way of knowing whether this reflected an uncertainty on their part about the nature of our relationship, a general lack of social skills or the fact that where they lived did not really feel like their own homes – certainly, the women I interviewed on hospital wards would not have felt like they could, and may well not have been allowed to, wander into the kitchen and put the kettle on whenever they felt like it.

Another way I tried to create an informal atmosphere was to allow the women to smoke in the office when they asked for permission to do so. Clearly, the fact that *I* was in a position to allow *them* to smoke indicates where the power lay. However, I personally dislike smoking and object to being in a small room with a smoker and I would usually tell the women that I did not like it. They almost always went ahead and smoked anyway, which I took as a positive sign in that they felt they had some control of the situation and were not behaving in a way to please me. I always wore casual clothes to interview the women (which, again, clearly distinguished me from the doctors or psychologists) and spoke to the women in a way which I felt was friendly, informal and on respectful and inclusive terms. The only exceptions to this were the few occasions when one or two women behaved in ways which I considered to be socially and personally unacceptable, such as shouting angrily at me (see p.118 for a discussion on dealing with difficult interview situations).

Anonymity and confidentiality

Anonymity and confidentiality are obviously as important for people with learning disabilities as for any other research subjects, but these can be difficult to explain. With regard to anonymity, people need to know that their names and any other identifying details will not be used in the dissemination of the research findings. But for people who do not read at all, or if they do, certainly do not read, or have any awareness that other people might read, the kinds of material research findings are likely to be reported in (journals, non-fiction books, conference reports), they may have very little idea what the researcher is actually talking about. In addition to this is the fact that whilst attempts at anonymity can and should be made, it can never be guaranteed.

Confidentiality can be easier to explain as it can be related more closely and concretely to the individual's situation – that is, the researcher can reassure someone by using actual people's names that their keyworker, fellow residents or their sexual partner will not find out what they have said. Wyngaarden (1981) gives a clever example of a researcher drawing a map of the country to show how far away the researcher was going with the research material and that no one close to the interviewee would see it. However, this would only work with those people with learning disabilities who understood that maps were symbolic representations of geographical distance and, clearly, not everyone has the capacity to understand this.

An important point to make regarding confidentiality is that researchers have to be clear themselves what they will keep confidential and what they will not, and this is not always an easy decision. The more personal and sensitive the topic, the more blurred the boundaries may become, but even researchers who interview people about what they might consider relatively safe topics can find themselves in difficulty over confidentiality. For example, a researcher asking people with learning disabilities about their preferred type of accommodation could quite easily hear from respondents that they did not like their group home because they were being abused there. The researcher would have to decide whether to act on that information (preferably with the co-operation of the individual who had disclosed it, but perhaps without it) or whether to merely record it as an interesting research finding.

Booth and Booth (1994), whilst acknowledging the stress for the researcher when they hear stories of individual suffering, assert that 'our position is that confidentiality must be upheld' (p.40). They go on to say that no researcher should be expected to bear this burden alone and describe the 'reference group' they set up for support. Researchers would use this group to anonymously present ethically difficult or distressing information that they had heard in their interviews. This seems a very appropriate course of action, although the fact that such information was presented anonymously to the reference group suggests that it was never intended that action might be taken. This still leaves the lone researcher with the burden of knowing exactly which individual was suffering. The Booths relate that they had to listen to interviewees talk about such distressing experiences as rape, incest and other child abuse. I assume that this refers to adult interviewees describing their own past experiences of such abuse and am left wondering what would have happened if one of their interviewees, inadvertently or otherwise, revealed that they were currently abusing their own child. This is by no means beyond the realms of possibility and surely would have challenged the Booths' assertion of always upholding confidentiality.

My position with regards to confidentiality was somewhat different from other researchers' because my research was carried out in the context of providing a sex education service to the women who had been referred to me for that purpose. As the majority of the interviews were carried out under the auspices of the Sex Education Team, I worked to the accepted confidentiality policy of that service. (As I had been a founder member of the team, I was well acquainted with the policy.) For those interviews not carried out under the umbrella of that team, I worked to the same principles anyway. This meant that the permission of all people with learning disabilities was sought to feedback a limited amount of information to key members of staff in order that ongoing support could be provided after the short-term intervention of sex education was over. If individuals gave their permission for this, which all the women in this study did (and which in my broader experience of working with approximately seventy women with learning disabilities happened in almost all circumstances), it was agreed with them which named members of staff the information would be shared with. If they refused permission for this sharing of personal information, they would be offered a completely confidential service. These, then, were the confidentiality arrangements I made with the women I interviewed for this study. However, it is worth noting that even if I had agreed complete confidentiality, there are circumstances in which I would have been prepared to break it – for example, if I was given reason to believe that the woman herself, or another named person, was in danger of imminent and serious harm. Breaking confidentiality in this way may well lead to the breakdown of trust in, and, therefore, the end to, the research and /or therapeutic relationship, but that would have to be accepted as the price to be paid – it is, as McLeod (1994) states, 'the basic moral imperative to respect and prevent harm to research participants' (p.172).

Informed consent

Despite the importance of it for research, until very recently (see Arscott *et al.* 1998; Stalker 1998; Swain, Heyman and Gillman 1998) there has been relatively little in the literature on interviewing people with learning disabilities on the issue of obtaining informed consent. Traditionally (e.g. Atkinson 1989; Booth and Booth 1994; Wyngaarden 1981), there were descriptions of the research project being explained and people with learning disabilities simply being asked, usually by a member of staff already known to them, if they would like to participate. This is the most obvious course of action and, indeed, it is hard to think of a better alternative. Nevertheless, it is a flawed approach for a number of reasons: first, the commonly recognised general compliance and acquiescence of many people with learning disabilities would lead them to consent rather than decline in most instances; second, being asked to participate in research by a known (and presumably trusted) member of staff may well increase their tendency to consent (although, interestingly, the Booths conclude the opposite); and, third, it assumes that, through a brief and simple description of the research project, people with learning disabilities, usually unfamiliar with the concept and activities of research, will have sufficient grasp of the information to really know what they are consenting to. It is my contention, and this is very rarely explored in the literature (see Swain, Heyman and Gillman 1998 for an exception), that it is one thing to consent to the face-to-face aspects of research – that is, consent to talking to an individual researcher – and it is quite another to consent to the hidden, or behind-the-scenes, aspects of research – that is, the researcher going away with your answers, analysing them, coming to conclusions about you and your situation (which you may not even understand, much less agree with) and then informing others what they have discovered about you and people like you. Obviously, the more significant the learning disability, the less insight people are going to have, or be able to develop, about the hidden aspects of research. The Booths, for example, working with more able people, observed that 'people were genuinely engaged by the idea that others might benefit from their experience. Perhaps, too, some were flattered by the prospect of featuring in a book' (1994, p.29). One of my interviewees (one of, if not the most, intellectually able) also had a good insight into what I was trying to achieve with my research and was keen to help others by telling me her experiences. Most of the other interviewees, I felt, had much less insight into why I was talking to them and what I was going to do with the information they gave me. I explained, as carefully and simply as I could, that, first, it was so that I could learn more about how women with learning disabilities experienced their sexual lives and, second, once I had learned more, I wanted to help other people understand and so would talk to people and write about what I had learned. This was so that we would then be able to give women better help and support with their relationships and with sex. Explained in this way, all the women I asked to participate agreed, although for the reasons described above and because of their general lack of familiarity with the written word, how professionals and staff are educated, how services operate, etc, I would question whether this amounts to genuinely informed consent (see also Swain, Heyman and Gillman 1998). Homan (1991) is one of the very few other writers who has provided a critique of the way the principle of obtaining informed consent is usually put into practice, especially with subjects whose ability to understand is compromised:

> A[n] assumption is that consenting subjects have a sufficient awareness of what they are disclosing....The point we make here refers rather to a differential vision of the social researcher and participants. The subject may have control over the release of raw data, but the researcher attaches a significance to these that untrained subjects may not apprehend...This differential intellectual capacity is not confined to the use of children as subjects. (p.92)

Perhaps a more controversial question to ask is whether genuinely informed consent for the whole research process is actually necessary. Clearly, people need to give consent to those parts of the research process they can understand and have some control over – that is, meeting and talking to the researcher, being recorded on tape, only answering certain questions. For the more hidden and longer term aspects of the research, which many people are unlikely to understand and have little or no control over, three possible courses of action present themselves. First, researchers could invest much more time and effort in describing and demonstrating, in as concrete a way as possible, exactly what it is people are being asked to consent to and what their involvement will be (Arscott *et al.* 1998). Second, people with learning disabilities themselves could be fully involved in all stages of the research design, data collection and analysis and dissemination (Minkes *et al.* 1995; Townsley 1995). Third, it could be accepted that some people with learning disabilities are not in a position to give informed consent and to develop ethical practice to proceed in the absence of this (Brown and Thompson 1997; Stalker 1998). These are not mutually exclusive options and much more work needs to be done in this whole area as all options involve a lot more time and effort for researchers. But all seem like more honest strategies than assuming, on the basis of a few words of explanation, that people with intellectual limitations and little access to the world of ideas are giving their considered and informed consent to the whole of a complex research process.

As well as creating more work for researchers, such an approach would also involve a shift in perspective amongst many people who sit on research ethics committees. My own experience, and that of other researchers who have tried to problematise the notion of informed consent (see Brown and Thompson 1997), is that ethics committees find this hard to take on board. Typically, they want assurances that informed consent will be obtained and they want to see evidence of consent, ideally by a signed consent form. They are not easily convinced that such evidence of consent is often meaningless. For this research study I went to two ethics committees, the first (at the NHS Trust) for permission to proceed (where no particular issue was made about informed consent) and the second (at my own department at the university) for general ethical guidance. This second committee recommended that all the women I interviewed should sign a consent form. I argued against this on the grounds that many of the women did not read well or at all and so it would be patronising to ask them to sign a piece of paper when they did not know exactly what was written on it and that it would have been extremely easy for me to get them to sign the form (or indeed anything else for that matter), given the perceived power and authority I, or anyone in my position, had. Although the ethics committee was sympathetic to (rather than totally convinced by) my argument that evidence of consent does not necessarily mean genuinely and freely given informed consent (Homan (1991) describes the signing of consent forms by subjects who do not fully understand as a 'thinly disguised indemnity principle' (p.93)), they were, nevertheless, adamant that evidence was necessary. We eventually agreed on a compromise whereby I would record the conversation I had with each woman, in which I would explain the research project, and her consent to participate would be recorded. However, on reflection, I was not happy with the compromise for two main reasons. First, all the women were assured by me, when I was seeking their permission to use the tape recorder, that I would never allow anyone else to hear the tape and, in fact, that I would not keep the recording after transcription. I felt that to say that one part of the tape would be treated differently to the rest would create confusion and possibly be anxiety-provoking. Second, given that I believe, as other researchers do (e.g. Booth and Booth 1994) that permission to record someone's voice must always be gained every time the tape recorder is used I could not quite work out the logistics of how I was meant to switch on the tape recorder to record the discussion in which I was to describe the research *before* the person had agreed to take part in it. In the event, because of the complications described above and because I was coming towards the end of the study (the ethics committee not having been in existence before then), I decided not to follow their recommendations. Swain, Heyman and Gillman (1998), in discussing research with people with learning disabilities, provide a coherent and convincing argument that ethical considerations are not easily or adequately addressed at one moment in time – that is, at the outset or when approaching ethics committees. Rather, they argue that ethics be seen as a 'continuous process of decision making' which runs through the whole research project, up to and including publication.

Methods

Putting research theory into practice

Putting methodological and ethical principles into practice, especially when working on research with people with learning disabilities, has frequently been described as a 'minefield' (Brown and Thompson 1997; Swain, Heyman and Gillman 1998). Nevertheless, it must be done. The research method I chose for this study was that of the semi-structured in-depth interview. The reason for that choice was that I did not consider any other research method to be as suitable. Based on my prior work and research experience in the field, I was starting from the premise that the only people who can tell a researcher how they experience their sexual lives are the individuals themselves – in the case of women with learning disabilities, other people, such as staff or carers, often simply do not know. Therefore, it was clear that I would need a form of enquiry which went directly to the individuals concerned. Questionnaires, a common form of enquiry into explicitly sexual matters (e.g. Hite 1976; Quilliam 1994), would not have been suitable because of the literacy problems faced by most people with learning disabilities. This meant that my research had to involve my talking directly to women with learning disabilities and the options were to do this on a group or individual basis. I had considerable experience in facilitating sex education groups for women with learning disabilities and had observed that, generally, the level of discussion was at a more superficial level than my one-to-one sessions with women of similar abilities who had had similar experiences. There is a suggestion that using focus groups can facilitate discussion that might be inhibited in the more intense situation of one-to-one work (Thompson 1996) but, although this sounds entirely feasible, there is, as yet, little evidence to substantiate this when discussing very personal matters with people with learning disabilities. Therefore, I felt that to maximise the chances of the women feeling comfortable enough to be open and honest, individual interviews would be the most appropriate research method.

I rejected the format of highly structured interviews because they restrict the interviewer to pre-set questions and do not allow for flexibility and follow-up discussion. Once again, based on my prior work and academic experience, I knew that such a format would not work well with people with learning disabilities. It is necessary to adapt one's language and sentence construction with different people with learning disabilities, depending on their levels of intellectual ability and communication skills. It would be impossible to construct one set of questions that would suit everybody – the questions would inevitably be too complex for some and patronisingly simple for others.

Just as highly structured interviews were judged to be inappropriate, so were completely unstructured ones. As explained earlier, open-ended questions often do not facilitate discussion amongst people with learning disabilities, who tend to give short answers and wait for the next question or not answer at all. For example, in this research one general open-ended question such as 'can you tell me about your sexual experiences?' would very likely elicit no response. This is not merely because my respondents had learning disabilities but because sex is a difficult thing for most people to talk about freely and at length.

It therefore seemed clear to me that semi-structured in-depth interviews were the most appropriate form of enquiry. The interviews had to be in-depth because time is necessary for both parties (but particularly the respondents) to develop trust and rapport. When the subject matter is as highly personal and essentially private as an individual's sexual experiences, brief or superficial investigations will not do. Another important reason for choosing the in-depth semi-structured interview related to the overall context of my role with the women. The semi-structured interview most closely matched the style of work I was already doing with the women – that is, individual educational and counselling sessions on a broad range of sexuality issues. In fact, I made every effort to attempt to make the active research phase of my work as similar as possible to the rest of the time we spent together. Aside from obvious advantages of consistency of approach, this was an ethical decision designed to cause minimal disruption to any woman who might want to decide half-way through the research interviews that she no longer wished to take part. She could then have continued to receive education and counselling from me without any abrupt switch in my manner or support. This happened in one case during this research. The only discernible difference between those sessions that counted as research and those which did not was the use of the tape recorder for the research sessions. This was a small dictaphone-type machine that was unobtrusive and which the women did not seem to feel inhibited by. This assessment is obviously from my perspective as researcher but is based on what the women said and did and none appeared bothered by the tape recorder. Most took up the offer to hear some of the interview on tape but, having heard what they sounded like on tape, few showed any interest in the tape recorder thereafter.

I did not impose any overall limit on the amount of time I spent with each woman, although each session was limited to a maximum of one hour (because it is hard to concentrate for longer than this and also because of the practicalities of daily life and work). There was no artificial limit set on the number of sessions I had with each woman and, in practice, it varied from approximately six to twenty weekly sessions, although not all of these would have been the interviews I used for research purposes. Clearly, working in this way is very time consuming and would, therefore, be seen by some researchers as a disadvantage. But, from my point of view, I felt it would have been counter-productive, as well as unethical, to try to rush the women. Some people with learning disabilities need a lot of time to think and speak and they deserve to be given that time and opportunity. Other people with learning disabilities speak a great deal, sometimes very quickly, in what seems quite a compulsive way. A lot of what they have to say seems, at first hearing, not to be very relevant to the topic of conversation. But sometimes it is and time needs to be spent 'sifting through' what is not relevant or important. Other people may talk in a way that is quite repetitive, but it is still important to listen to them carefully – repetitive and/or echolalic speech by people with learning disabilities may not be because they cannot help it (as is often assumed) but because they are trying to say something important and no-one is listening (Sinason 1994).

I made efforts to be true to the principles of feminist research methodology I mentioned earlier by treating my respondents as women with interesting and important things to say and not merely as sources of research material with whom contact would cease once sufficient material had been generated. But, obviously, there were limits – however much they felt they had to say, the women could not go on talking forever. I had to use my feelings as a guide when to intervene. If a woman was talking at great length about topics not related to the research or my broader work agenda, I did try to intervene – either to stop her talking temporarily (so I could get a chance to say something) or to bring her back to the topic in question.

Another potential disadvantage of my chosen research method is that it does rely almost entirely on first-hand accounts from those involved and, therefore, relies for its validity on people being truthful. Other researchers on sexual matters have had to face the question of whether their respondents are telling the truth: Kinsey, Pomeroy and Martin (1948) felt that an experienced researcher would be able to tell from the way a respondent spoke and from their body language whether they were being truthful. He also checked the consistency of interviews taken at different points in time and cross-checked accounts given by spouses; Schaefer (1973) relied on a conviction that as people voluntarily taking part in research, subjects had no need to lie about or distort their accounts. Other researchers – for example, Hite (1976) – do not address the issue.

There is no reason to think that people with learning disabilities are likely to be any less truthful than other people. But sexuality is an issue that often causes people anxiety and confusion and it is a 'loaded' subject in that it is value laden and this leads many people to want to give a certain impression of themselves and others. However, rather than dismissing individuals' testimonies as inherently unreliable on those grounds, my approach was to take answers to individual questions in the context of the *whole* account and build up a picture of what is happening for that individual. For instance, when enquiring into sexual abuse, all researchers need to be aware that some people (with and without learning disabilities) are reluctant to admit that they have been abused or that men they had meaningful relationships with would perpetrate abuse against them (Kelly 1996). Therefore, the somewhat stark questions 'have you ever been abused?' or 'has anyone ever forced you to do something sexual you didn't want to do?' may well elicit the answer 'no'. However, supplementary questions, such as what kind of sex the woman likes and dislikes and what kind of sex she actually has on a regular basis, can be very revealing. This is also true of questions about who makes the decisions about sex, who wants it the most, who likes it the most, who experiences pleasure or pain from which activities. These questions allow the researcher to build up a detailed picture and can tap into experiences and feelings that are otherwise easily overlooked. As I explained earlier, I took time to reflect back to the women the things they had said, to check with them that I had received their information accurately. This is not quite what is meant in the literature by 'respondent validation' (Silverman 1993) as this seems to imply taking the whole body of one's findings and analysis back to the research subjects for their critical reflection. This is not something I attempted with the women in this study, for practical and methodological reasons. I am not aware of examples where this had happened with people with learning disabilities, although the small but growing number of research projects which involve people with learning disabilities at all stages (Young 1996) stand the most chance of doing this successfully. Indeed, the literature relating to people with learning disabilities does suggest 'checking out' findings and analysis by returning with it to the research participants (Stalker 1998). However, this does presuppose that after some considerable time (quite easily a year or two later in the case of big projects) participants would have an interest in, and accurate memory of, what they originally said and meant.

In addition to the possibility that certain individuals might not be truthful, or might be forgetful, there is also the complex matter of what it is possible or socially acceptable to say about sexual matters. It is not a simple question of people telling the truth or untruths. Rather there are questions about what does the truth *mean* in relation to 'telling sexual stories' (Plummer 1995). Individuals' experiences are moderated through public and highly gendered discourses about what is and what is not acceptable and appropriate. The lack of, and need for, positive sexual discourses for women is raised in Chapter Six.

However, it would not be true to say that *all* my information for this research came directly from the women themselves, although certainly most of it did. I was also able to use the knowledge I built up over a number of years about the environments the women lived in and the other people they associated with. This knowledge was often useful to substantiate or (occasionally) cast doubt on something a woman had said. Triangulation, the comparison of data for corroboration, is commonly cited in the literature as being an appropriate way to attempt to validate findings (McLeod 1994; Silverman 1993). In particular, it is noted that to be an 'insider' or 'empirically literate' (Roseneil 1993) – that is, already familiar with a system or environment – gives a researcher a considerable advantage in that one has a 'built-in truth check' (Riemer 1977, p.474 cited in Roseneil 1993).

Sometimes, the fact that I had broader knowledge of the circumstances of the women's lives, plus all my other experience of working with a much larger group of women with learning disabilities on sexuality issues, meant that I could make the inferences that ethnographers have to make. For example, in this study one woman told me that she had stayed with various non-disabled men in their flats when she would otherwise have been temporarily homeless. Although she did not say it directly and may not even have realised it on a conscious level, I inferred from other things she said about the men that they probably expected sexual favours in return for providing a roof over her head. I felt confident to make this inference on the basis that my wider experience had shown me many examples of non-disabled men sexually exploiting women with learning disabilities in situations like this and no examples of acts of generosity and kindness expecting nothing in return. Of course, I have to, and do, allow for the fact that my inferences may be wrong. I have sought to present my findings in such a way that those who wish to take issue with my inferences and conclusions can demonstrate how and why I am wrong.

Data analysis

Because of the nature of the data and the investigation, a multi-staged narrative analysis was undertaken (Stevens 1994). The first stage was to transcribe each interview, then read and re-read each one separately until I was familiar with each woman, what she had said and how she had said it. For the second stage, I reduced the data by producing a summary of each woman's account, drawing out key points and any significant features of her telling of it. In the third stage I went back to the original data set and reorganised it so that for each question I had all seventeen women's answers mapped out together. I was then able to broadly categorise the responses onto a chart, a separate one for each question. I then took each category in turn and returned to the data to interpret what the women had said and used their own words to explain or strengthen particular points and/or the overall picture. The fourth stage of analysis involved examining basic themes, patterns of shared experience and diversity.

This method of data analysis, sometimes referred to as the 'editing style' is considered to be particularly appropriate when the goal of the research is 'subjective understanding, exploration, and/or generation of new insights/hypotheses and when scant knowledge already exists' (Miller and Crabtree 1992, p.20). As such, it seemed entirely suited to this research project. It is a lengthy and, therefore, time-consuming method of data analysis and, for all the researcher's efforts, the end result may appear relatively straightforward. However, this is at least part of the point of it: 'Parts are strung together to make new wholes – simplicity is sought beneath the complexity' (Reinharz 1983, p.182). The alternative would be to give a purely quantitative account of qualitative data or to leave the reader overwhelmed with huge amounts of data to examine and interpret for themselves. As I have criticised Hite's sexological research on both these accounts (see p.27), this was clearly something I wished to avoid myself.

Reciprocity and identification

The Booths (1994), like many feminist researchers (e.g. Oakley 1981; Phoenix 1994), emphasise the need for researchers to be prepared to answer personal questions as well as ask them. Ferrarotti (1981) has stated that if researchers want intimate knowledge from interviewees, the trade-off is to be reciprocally known just as thoroughly. This may be so in theory but I would suggest that it would take particularly confident research subjects to ask as much of the researcher as is asked of them. Although I was prepared to, and in fact always did, answer any personal questions put to me by the women I interviewed, in reality few personal questions were asked. Additionally, at the end of every interview I openly acknowledged the one-sidedness of the situation – that is, that I had asked them lots of questions and explicitly offered each woman an opportunity to ask me anything she liked. This opportunity was almost always declined, indicating either that they were not curious about my personal or sexual life or that, despite my efforts to create an atmosphere of equality, they did not feel able to ask me such things as I had asked them. When the women did ask me personal questions, they were about whether I engaged in specific sexual activities and this was a sobering reminder that even when it is your job to talk and write about sex all day, as mine has been for several years now, it is quite a different matter to talk about your own sex life. More usually, however, the women asked for personal information that seemed to help them 'place' me as a woman (Cotterill 1992; Finch 1984) – for example, whether I was married or living with someone, whether I had children, etc. At the time of the research, I was not married or living with a partner and I did not have children, but I did have occasional sexual relationships with men. This meant that my sexual lifestyle was similar to theirs in some respects. I realise, of course, that I am vastly more privileged in many ways but I was closer to them in this respect than many of the other non-disabled women they would have come into contact with – for example, staff and carers. Most of these other women would have been married/cohabiting, most with children and, even if they were not, these assumptions are often made by people with learning disabilities and go unchallenged by staff members (McCarthy and Thompson 1994b).

Whilst reciprocity in revealing personal information is usually only seen in positive terms, it does have a down side in that it can lead to research participants revealing more about themselves than they otherwise would, and more than they perhaps should, in certain circumstances (Swain, Heyman and Gillman 1998). Whether or not the women I interviewed felt more inclined to open up to me because they felt we may have had things in common is hard to tell. But it did seem to be the case that with some women, at least, revealing personal information about myself could lead to the woman identifying with me, or me with her, and this definitely led to a feeling of connection between us. For example, one woman said that she found herself 'giving in' to men sexually – that is, having sex with them when she did not really feel like it herself – because to assert herself would risk causing a fuss, having a row. She was unhappy about this but, nevertheless, found herself doing it over and over again. To let her know that I understood what she meant, I said that I had done the same thing myself and thought that probably lots of women had. The following discussion no longer focused on her as an individual but was an inclusive discussion about women as 'we' and 'us'.

At other times, however, revealing personal information could have the opposite effect and lead a woman to position me as being different from her, as the following exchange shows (in all the dialogues in this book, the initials 'MM' refer to the author):

MC: Has any man ever asked you to have it up the anus?

MM: No.

MC: If they did, would you do it?

MM: No, I don't think so.

MC: So you're not soft then, not like me.

MM: Well, that's not always true. I have done things I wish I hadn't but I do try to stand up for myself. It's not easy though.[1]

In my last few sentences here I try to encourage some identification between us, not least because it was true but also because I did not want to risk her putting herself down by seeing me as a woman who was necessarily, in all circumstances, more skilled or assertive.

In both my research interviews and my wider work experience I have tried to let the women know that I am 'on their side'. Finch (1984) suggests this is consistent with major traditions in sociological research and Cocks and Cockram (1995) suggest it is essential for any research which aims to improve the circumstances of the lives of people with learning disabilities: 'The researcher must have a sensitivity and democratic identification with the people who are the subjects of the investigation, the oppressed' (p.34.). I do have a genuine feeling of concern for, and solidarity with, the women with learning disabilities with whom I work. Therefore, it is not an attitude I felt obliged to adopt for the purposes of gaining access to the women's lives in order to do the research. Because of this, conducting the research has had an emotional impact on me (Moran-Ellis 1996). I have often felt great sadness and rage at what many of the women have been through. Occasionally, there have been moments of humour and joy but these have largely been as a result of the personal interaction between the women and myself rather than my reactions to what they have told me about their lives. As will become apparent in the next chapter, the overall tone of what the women have had to say about their sexual lives is negative and depressing. As the researcher, I have been enmeshed in this rather grim picture for a number of years and it

1   The initials used to refer to individual women are fictitious.

has depressed me too. However, it has not always been the predictable things that have upset me most: one of the worst moments for me was being asked to sign the plaster cast of a woman who had broken her arm and seeing the words 'retard' and 'spastic' written there by non-disabled students at her college, people she considered to be her friends. Realising later that I felt more upset about this small act of cruelty than when other women told me about being raped, I then felt guilty at having got my priorities all wrong. It must also be said that, along with the feelings of sadness, I have taken inspiration from the strength and resilience of many of the women and this has helped me to retain a sense of balance and perspective.

It is often stated, and generally accepted as being true, that to be actively involved in sexuality or sexual health work, workers have to be comfortable with their own sexuality (see, for example, Krajicek 1982; Lee 1996). I have never been exactly sure what is meant by this and nobody ever seems to elaborate on it. All I can say for myself is that I am in no doubt that my sexuality affects the work I do and the work I do affects my sexuality. As I have reflected elsewhere (McCarthy 1991), like many other women, with and without learning disabilities, I have had both positive and negative sexual experiences with men. These are not just things that happen to the subjects of my research, they are a part of my life and I do not pretend to be objective or neutral in any discussion about heterosexual relations. What I have done in this research is different from a lot of other research about non-sexual topics and different from much of the research my colleagues in the learning disability field are engaged in – for example, investigating how people with learning disabilities feel about their residential or day services. Researchers of such topics rarely have any personal experiences of their own to compare, contrast or reflect on.

My influence as a researcher

To complete this section on methods, it is important to reflect on what effect I would have had on the women I interviewed – both in terms of the factors mentioned above and also more broadly. The question needs to be posed as to how much I would have influenced them because, as a member of staff, I was clearly in a position of power. Also, because of my informal approach in terms of the way I dressed and the way I spoke and treated the women, I know that coming to see me was a different experience for the women than, for example, being interviewed or counselled by their consultant psychiatrist or psychologist. The women themselves said as much and from the few such interviews with other professionals which I had directly observed I knew this to be the case. The women I interviewed, with one or two exceptions, seemed to like me very much and none appeared to be afraid that I might use my power within the system(s) to affect them adversely. These observations are based on what the women themselves said about talking to me:

JM: You're easy to talk to.

EY: I like talking to you.

MH: It's good coming to see you.

However, I was also aware that, for at least one of the women, there was a good, practical reason for her wanting to spend time with me. She shared her learning disability service with her ex-boyfriend who was harassing her:

I like coming to talk to you because it gets me out of his way, he can't aggravate me then. (JR)

Given the positive relationship that usually existed between the women and myself, then, it would make sense to assume that the women wanted to please rather than offend me with their responses to my questions. Therefore, the potential existed, as in any such relationship, that I could get the responses I was looking for from the women rather than what they really felt or did. But for the women to give me what they considered to be the 'right' response, they would have to work out first what I wanted to hear. What I *wanted* to hear was about happy, mutual, pleasurable sex lives which contributed to the women's sense of well-being. What I *expected* to hear (on the basis of my own prior work, but also the vast body of feminist knowledge on the area) was about a lot of negative and abusive sexual experiences. The fact that I have heard what I expected to hear means that I must question whether I asked (consciously or sub-consciously) leading questions to get the required answers. Not surprisingly, I think I did not. The research was carried out so I could gain a PhD. My work was supervised and I was, in any case, aware of the rigorous academic standards required of research at this level. Consequently, I made efforts not to ask what could be construed as leading questions and I restrained myself from expressing the full horror of what I felt when the women described abuse, although obviously expressing sympathy and understanding when appropriate. Inevitably there were moments when I did give my own personal opinion on certain subjects, which could be interpreted as me trying to influence the women, except that I made sure I only gave the women my opinions after they had given me theirs. For example, when discussing men's use of pornography with one woman, I did tell her my views on that, but only after she had told me hers first, so I would not be influencing what she had to say for the research. Similarly, in a discussion with another woman on the reasons why men rape (see p.173), I do give an opinion, but in response to hers, not before it. Therefore, I am as confident as I can be that I did not influence the women's responses to specific questions as they were asked. However, like every other researcher, I have no way of knowing whether any of the women who participated in this study might have altered their views in line with mine over the longer term or, indeed, altered their responses to subsequent questions in line with what they may have imagined mine to be.

It is also important to note that, at certain times, both during the research interviews and during my other contacts with the women, I *was* actively trying to influence them. After all, the research interviews were being conducted in the context of my being paid to provide a service to the women. I was meant to influence them with regard to recognising that they had choices, in helping them to become more assertive, in practising safer sex, etc. I was not meant to, and do not believe I did, influence their individual sexual preferences or encourage them to tell me things, positive or negative, which were not the case.

Managing difficult situations

It would be true to say that, for the vast majority of the time I spent with the seventeen women I interviewed, the process was largely unproblematic. But there were also some difficult moments. In one session, when I was explaining to a woman what and where the clitoris was, she wanted me to check, there and then, whether she had one. I explained I could not do that as I was not a doctor or nurse and, therefore, was not allowed to look at people's bodies. She dismissed this as a good enough reason and continued with her pleas that I check and started to undress. After much protesting on my part and informing her that I would leave the room if she undressed, she finally accepted that I could not do what she wanted. We agreed on a compromise whereby I gave her the sex education picture showing where the clitoris was and she agreed to examine herself in the bathroom later, with the help of her female keyworker if necessary. In another session, a different woman, who could be quite volatile, suddenly turned her anger on me in a very personal way. She appeared to misinterpret something I said and completely lost her temper with me, shouting aggressively at me at the top of her voice for several minutes. I tried to de-escalate the situation by remaining calm and firm until she cooled down enough for me to explain that I was not prepared to accept such behaviour from her and I ended the session, making sure she understood she could come back again. When she returned the following week, she apologised for her outburst and it never happened again. Both the above situations were moments when my wish to treat the women on respectful, equal and inclusive terms would have been temporarily suspended. My tone of voice and what I said would have become more authoritative in an effort to gain some control over a situation which looked like it might pose a personal threat or, at the very least, was decidedly risky.

Not all the difficult or unusual situations were unpleasant, however. Some were just odd. When I was interviewing one woman, she suddenly stuck her arms out straight in a kind of crucifixion pose and held them there:

MM: Why have you got your arms out like that?

TC: Because I've got some soreness.

MM: Are you going to keep them like that?

TC: Yes. [Laughs] All right I won't if you don't want me to.

MM: It's not that I don't want you to, but it does look a bit funny.

[Both laugh]

At the risk of stigmatising people with learning disabilities, it is hard to imagine similar situations to the ones described above happening in research interviews with non-disabled people. However, they could happen and, therefore, any researcher would do well to expect the unexpected and be prepared.

Conclusion

By choosing the appropriate research method for the task and getting the overall context right (i.e. offering counselling, support and advice where necessary), it has been my experience in this study that many women with learning disabilities are able to give clear and coherent accounts of their sexual lives – not only factual accounts of what happens but also what they feel about what happens and what sense they make of it. Often, women with learning disabilities do not have many opportunities to discuss sexual matters (see p.134). However, given time, encouragement and respect, I found that most of the women were willing to share their experiences, thoughts and feelings. Sensitive interviewing, in the context of offering advice and support, can facilitate this.

CHAPTER FOUR

The Sexual Lives of Women with Learning Disabilities
Research Findings

Introduction

The women whose experiences are represented in this study were the first 17 women referred to me for sex education/counselling who fitted the criteria I had set for inclusion in the research study. These criteria were that:

- the women had to have had some sexual experience with at least one other person
- they had to be verbally articulate enough to be able to talk about these experiences
- they had to agree to discuss their experiences with me.

There were no other criteria. All interviews took place between the end of 1992 and 1996. The 17 women who took part in this research study reported experiences and expressed views which were very broadly representative of the much larger number of approximately 70 women with learning disabilities with whom I have worked on sexuality issues over the past eight or so years (McCarthy 1996b). At different points throughout this chapter I highlight where there are any significant differences or similarities between the sub-group of 17 and the bigger group of 70.

Of the 17 women, 8 had their sexual experiences predominantly in learning disability hospitals and 7 had their experiences predominantly in community settings. Two women had sexual experiences both in hospital and the community. Five of the 10 women who had spent time in hospitals had been, or were on, locked wards. This did not mean that they were supervised at all times, however, as all had varying amounts of unsupervised time in the hospital grounds. Being on a locked ward was an indication of a diagnosis of an additional mental health problem and being detained under Section Three (treatment order) of the Mental Health Act 1983. Of the 9 women who lived or had lived predominantly in the community, 6 lived in small group homes run by social services or voluntary organisations, one woman lived alone in her own home which she had shared with her mother until her mother's death and two women had lived in a variety of settings, including their parental homes, in the flats of men they were in relationships with and in group homes.

The ages of the women were between nineteen and fifty-five, with roughly one-third being in their twenties, one-third in their thirties and one-third in their forties. Consequently, the particular needs and experiences of the very young and very old are not included in this study. However, the ages of the women who are included could be seen as broadly representative of most sexually active adults with learning disabilities – there is evidence to suggest that when a sex education/counselling service is available to adults with learning disabilities, most referrals are of people in their twenties, thirties and forties (McCarthy 1996b).

All interviews were carried out in learning disability services in two counties of South-East England. As the service users in these areas are overwhelmingly white British people, this is reflected in the sample of women in this study. All 17 women were white; 16 of them were English and one was Irish, although she had lived in England for most of her life. The cultural homogeneity of this group is a reflection of the referrals made to the sex education team where most of this work was conducted, where 92 per cent of referrals were of white British people (McCarthy 1996b).

In my wider sex education and counselling experience with women with learning disabilities I have only had the opportunity to work with four Black British women. Their experiences and the ways in which they related them did not differ in any discernible way from those of many of the white women I have worked with. However, as I have remarked elsewhere, I do not consider myself particularly skilled or experienced in drawing those factors out (McCarthy 1996a). Added to this is the fact that, as a white woman, I may not be the most appropriate person to facilitate such discussion with Black women. It is hard to be sure about this as some research suggests that the skills and approach of workers is more significant than being of the same cultural background as clients (d'Ardenne and Mahtani 1989; see Phoenix 1994 for a fuller discussion of this issue). Nevertheless, the need for Black and ethnic minority workers to support service users and for all service providers to provide culturally sensitive attention to the sexuality needs of Black service users is highlighted in the literature (Baxter 1994; Malhotra and Mellan 1996).

The levels of learning disability of the 17 women interviewed for this study ranged from very mild/borderline to moderate/severe, with two-thirds being towards the more mild end of the spectrum. This is a reflection of the fact that in order to take part in a study which relied on verbal communication, the women had to have a relatively high level of understanding and verbal skills. However, it also reflects the fact that most referrals for sex education tend to be of the more able people and this in itself is a reflection of the fact that (excluding masturbation and sexual abuse) there is a correlation between higher levels of ability and sexual activity (McCarthy 1996b).

Only two of the women had recognisable syndromes related to their learning disability; both had chromosomal disorders, one had Down's Syndrome and one had Prader-Willi Syndrome. Five of the 17 women had additional mental health problems; one with a formal diagnosis of 'personality disorder', but most with a more general description of emotional and/or behavioural disturbance.

Research findings

Whether the women enjoyed their sexual activity

The first questions the women were asked were designed to open up the subject area and to give a general impression of how they felt about their sexual activity, which I would then follow up with more specific questions afterwards. At this early stage, then, the women were asked whether they liked having sex and to elaborate, where possible, on what it was they did or did not like. If this seems like a rather tall order for the very beginning of an interview, it should be remembered that this 'interview phase' of my work with the women came some way into my overall relationship with them. In effect, I would usually already have had several, and, at the very least, one or two sessions (each lasting approximately thirty minutes to an hour) with them so that we could get to know each other, explain what my work was about and generally build rapport. So, although it may appear on paper (see appendix for interview questions) that I sat down, said hello and then proceeded to ask 'do you like having sex?', this was far from the truth! As I make clear in Chapter Three, my intention was never to stick to a rigid and pre-set interview schedule. As will become apparent from the extracts of discussions quoted in this chapter, at times, my responses to the women were sympathetic and, at times, my questions were going off at a tangent to follow up on something interesting a woman had said but which was not necessarily within the focus of this research. In short, my research was very much rooted in the context of my wider relationships with the women.

The women's responses to the general question of whether they liked sex varied from very positive to very negative. Eight women were very negative and one was mostly negative, accounting for over half the whole sample:

> FM: I don't like the sex. It feels absolutely awful.
>
> MM: In what part of you does it feel awful?
>
> FM: If it was to feel inside of me, I think 'Oh no, I don't want that'. But I like kissing on the mouth.

> No, I don't like it at all. (GJ)

> The whole thing is horrible. (MH)

One woman was fairly neutral:

> [hesitatingly] I don't *mind* it, but not all the time, not all the time, like every night, because you get fed up. (BN)

Four women said that whether they liked sex or not depended on a variety of factors, such as whether they experienced physical pain and /or men treated them roughly:

> EY: Well if they're not rough it's all right. Well I always think that if anyone has sex they should go a bit more gentle, not like a dartboard … I'll tell what some men do, if they don't get your body, they attack you.
>
> MM: Yes, that can happen. What do you mean 'like a dartboard'?
>
> EY: Pushing themselves into you hard, you know, going mad…I don't like it like that, M. [boyfriend] does it like that
>
> MM: If the men are gentle, what is it you like about sex?
>
> EY: Well, it's nature, it's lovable and it makes a woman of you.

One woman (DY) said that sex was best if it involved love, which for her it often didn't, although it sometimes did, and one woman (GN) said she only liked sex with her boyfriend and then only if 'he did it' a certain way and these conditions were sometimes met and sometimes not.

Two women were mostly positive about their experiences, albeit with some reservations:

> I like doing it because I want to…depends on seeing what sort of man he is. (TM)

> I do like it when R. [boyfriend] does it to me, the front way. (GN)

Only one woman (TY) was very positive. Unfortunately for the research, she was one of the least intellectually able and least communicative, so it was not possible to find out much in the way of detail. However she expressed in simple and clear terms the fact that she liked what she did.

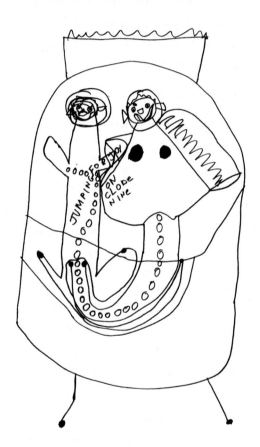

Figure 4.1

As an indirect way of gauging whether and how much the women enjoyed their sexual activity, they were asked to contemplate whether they would miss it if, for some reason, they had to stop. As this was a hypothetical question, a couple of the women found it too difficult and either misinterpreted it (thinking I was saying she should stop) or gave two inherently contradictory answers. But most women did understand. Six said they would miss sex, although one of these was clear that it was, in fact, the reward she would miss and not the sex itself – 'I'd miss the money...I only do it for what I can get out of it' (GJ).

Nine women said they would not miss sex, five of them being very emphatic about this. Interestingly almost half the nine women who said they would not miss sex had been amongst those who had previously expressed at least some positive feelings about it (see above). It is difficult to interpret this clearly but it implies that even where there were some positive aspects, these were not sufficient to make them want to continue. In addition, two women specifically mentioned having children at this point, either as a reason to continue having sex 'I wonder what the children will look like' (TM) or to note that giving up sex did not necessarily mean having to give up the possibility of having children 'You can always adopt children' (DO).

Who the women had sex with

None of the women said that she had ever had any sexual contact with another woman. Therefore, all the information in this study relates to heterosexual encounters and relationships. However, for the women's views on sex between women, see pages 130–132. There was a wide range of contexts for the women's sexual activity, ranging from one woman who had had one sexual partner to a number of women who had had many partners. (The word 'partner' feels like a very unsatisfactory term as it implies a mutuality that, as will become apparent in this chapter, was very often conspicuous only by its absence. However, for the lack of a better term, it will have to suffice.)

The single most common context for the women's sexual activity (relating to six of the seventeen) was to have sex only within an established relationship with men they identified as boyfriends. However, there was considerable variety even within this one category – one woman had had only one boyfriend for a few months, another had had the same boyfriend for several years and another had had several boyfriends one after the other. Almost as common as the above was for women to have sex predominantly with their boyfriends but also *occasionally* with other men who they were not in relationships with. These were either a variety of men with learning disabilities in the same service or repeatedly with one particular man. A variation on this pattern was one woman who had sex *regularly* with a number of casual partners (including strangers) as well as with established boyfriends. Three of the women had had sex with a variety of casual partners only and not with boyfriends. One of these women expressed regret that she could not find a boyfriend and considered what she was doing to be a 'second-best' option. Two of the women had arrangements whereby they had one long-standing and regular sexual partner who was not their boyfriend. In one case the man was actually the boyfriend of the woman's best friend and in the other the woman had her own boyfriend with whom she did not have a sexual relationship.

Five of the women explicitly said that they had sex with men who did not have learning disabilities. It is highly probable from the circumstances described by some of the other women that they also had had sex with non-disabled men, although they did not necessarily identify them as such. Sometimes, the women picked up on obvious signifiers or clues by which they determined whether a man had learning disabilities or not:

> EY: I've been with outside men.
>
> MM: How do you know they're outside men?
>
> EY: 'Cos they come in by car.

Men who do not have learning disabilities actively seeking out sexual encounters with women with learning disabilities has been noted from the early days of my work in this field (McCarthy 1993) and in other people's work (for example, Chenoweth 1996). Sometimes, ongoing relationships might be formed and, indeed, long-term partnerships and marriages do take place (see Chapter Two for further discussion). However, sometimes it was clear that the women were entering into purely sexual encounters:

> MM: How do you get on with the outside men?
>
> TY: They don't say anything, they don't talk to me.
>
> MM: Not at all?
>
> TY: No.

The women's perceptions of how men experienced sex with them

Unlike many men with learning disabilities, who, because they are focused on their own needs seem unaware of the needs of others (Gardiner, Kelly and

Wilkinson 1996) and, consequently, often do not know whether women like having sex with them, all but one of my interviewees knew (or, perhaps, more accurately, *thought* they knew) how their male sexual partners felt about having sex with them. These sixteen women all thought that the men liked it: six of these women were very sure about this, nodding their heads and using an emphatic tone of voice to accompany their verbal answers; nine others gave less marked, albeit still clear, responses; and one women said that generally men did like it but some appeared not to. Interestingly, one of the ways this woman thought she could tell if the men did not like sex was their use of physical violence – 'they try to hit you' (EY). But this was also a way the men expressed themselves if they *did* like sex and the women tried to prevent them – 'they beat you up' (EY). The way she distinguished between these acts of violence was by interpreting how the men were behaving more generally – that is, if they did not like the sex 'they lean away' (EY) whereas if they did 'they put their arms around you' (EY). Quite why some men were engaging in sex when they did not appear to be enjoying it was not clear. Presumably, it could have been something to do with changing their minds once they had started, something about the environment which upset them – for example, fear of being caught or observed – or not finding themselves sexually aroused. It is impossible to know. However, my wider work (McCarthy and Thompson 1992; McCarthy 1996b) in this field does not suggest that men routinely engage in sexual contact with women which the men neither want nor enjoy and does suggest that the men usually have the control to begin and end sexual encounters as they see fit. (See p.203 for further discussion.)

The women in this study seemed quite skilled at 'reading' the men's behaviour towards them – that is, they made what seem quite reasonable assumptions from what the men said and did. A number of the women, therefore, deduced that the men did like having sex with them because the men initiated it ('You can tell they want it, because they're all over you [laughs], kissing you and that, they're all over you' (BN)) or because the men came back for more or said they wanted sex again ('he used to keep on about it' (MH)). In only one case did a woman report that men specifically expressed appreciation for her body. However, this was tinged with some sadness and confusion for her because the men made what could be considered 'stock' or 'standard' remarks about women's sexual body parts but which, in fact, did not relate specifically to her – 'I don't know why they say about my breasts when I haven't got any' (MC). This woman had

Prader-Willi Syndrome and the underdevelopment of secondary sexual characteristics in people with this condition is common (Greenswag 1987).

However, it is also true that the women did not generally express much appreciation for the men's bodies either. In fact, only two comments were made about men's bodies throughout all the interviews: one women said she liked men to have a smooth, rather than a hairy, chest and another said she did not like men to have big penises because, as she very plainly put it, 'The bigger they are the more the fucking worse pain it is' (MC).

Masturbation

The women were asked whether they masturbated and, if they did, how this experience compared to having sex with men. In addition, whether they masturbated or not, women were asked generally what they thought about it – that is, whether they considered it an acceptable thing to do. Two women avoided the questions completely – one changed the subject to one loosely related to sexual matters (whether a blood test was needed to confirm pregnancy) and the other changed the subject completely (to her next meal). As such blatant avoidance was very unusual, I took these responses as clear signs that the women were uncomfortable with the subject and I respected that – that is, I did not press them to return to the topic.

Of the remaining fifteen women, the responses were divided equally into three categories: those who were quite definite that they did not masturbate and who had strong negative feelings about it ('I think it's rude, disgusting and vulgar' (FM), 'I never play with myself, so don't say I do, 'cos I don't, so there!' (TC)); those who said that they didn't masturbate themselves but who did not particularly express disapproval ('I suppose that's all right' (KN)); and those who tentatively said that they did masturbate now or had done so in the past ('[Smiling] I can't tell you. I used to when I was little' (GJ)). None of the women readily or confidently reported that they masturbated, despite my efforts to assure them that I considered it a perfectly normal and positive activity, something most women did. Of the five women who said they had masturbated, only two ventured a comparison of it in relation to heterosexual activity – one said that it was just different and one said that it gave her better feelings in her body than having sex with men did. Incidentally, this was the same woman who was unreservedly positive about her sexual activity with men (see above).

Two women expressed the belief that a woman could cause herself physical harm through masturbation – one thought it would cause sores and the other a more general injury which she likened to an incident when she had bled after having sex with a man:

MM: Is it [masturbation] wrong for men and women?

EY: For women because they can injure themselves. If they put their hand up the front and keep rubbing themselves, they might injure their vagina or something like that. I tell you something that happened to me, no word of a lie, when my ex-boyfriend used to interfere with me when I was on the other way, he made me pour with blood and I had to stop on the ward. The nurse done her nut and kept me in and told him to go away.

Two other women expressly said that it was wrong for women to masturbate because it could upset men: 'men would think it was funny, it would put them off' (MC); 'A man might see you...he'd have the shock of his life' (GN). When asked if, for instance, they thought women members of staff would masturbate, there were incredulous or shocked tones of voice when most of the women said no or that they did not know. One woman clearly said she thought only male staff would do it:

MM: But do you think people like staff do it?

FM: They can [laughs]... D. [male staff] would, R.[male staff] would...

MM: What about any of the women?

FM: Only the men would do it.

About one-third of the women referred to men's masturbation and they generally viewed this more positively, understanding it in the context of men needing to 'relieve' themselves – one woman, giving the example of a particular man, said 'R. gets these feelings and he has to go into the bathroom and get it over with' (KN); another took masturbation by men to be a sign of them actively wanting sex. For women, she saw things quite differently:

MC: ...men do it a lot if they feel sexually inclined towards a woman and they can't get one, but for women it's not a good idea, even if they're in bed, because it doesn't prove anything and it's wrong to do it.

MM: Is it wrong for men to masturbate?

MC: No because they'd like a woman to be in their life and they haven't got one. Masturbating is a good sign that they get those feelings, that they get urges.

MM: So men get sexual urges?

MC: Yes.

MM: Do you think women get sexual urges?

MC: No.

MM: Why not?

MC: The only sexual urges a woman can have is if a fella takes her to have sex. Otherwise they haven't got any.

My wider experience of talking to women with learning disabilities about sexual matters indicates that it is not unusual for the women to hold more positive views about masturbation for men than they do for themselves and to ascribe this to the notion of men's sexual urges (McCarthy 1993). It seems unlikely that the women would have come to this conclusion by themselves. Rather, I would suggest that the women have been given messages about the 'male sexual imperative' (Jackson 1984). It is possible that this view might be directly or indirectly imparted from staff, the media or other sources. One thing is certain, that it sometimes comes directly from men themselves:

> I've got a boyfriend and if I can't go out with him, and he's hard up for sex and would like a good session, he goes into the toilet – I know because he's told me – and does this [mimes male masturbation] (MC).'

Sex between women

None of the women reported any personal experience of sex with another woman. From the much larger group of approximately 70 women with learning disabilities I have worked with over the years, only one woman has discussed having sexual feelings for other women. This woman did not want to talk about it at all but the discussion was initiated and sustained by me as she had made abusive sexual advances towards other women with learning disabilities. Staff had also reported to me in my role as sex education worker that two women with learning disabilities were seen kissing intimately. In this instance there were no suggestions of any inappropriate behaviour and, as neither of the women chose to raise the subject with me, it was, therefore, not discussed. Aside from these very few women, lesbian sexuality has not otherwise appeared to be an interest or issue in the lives of the vast majority of women with learning disabilities I have met, something which the (admittedly sparse) literature on the topic confirms (see p.204 for further discussion on lesbian sexuality).

The women in this study were asked what they thought about sexual relationships between women. Only one expressed anything close to a positive view: 'It's up to them, it's their life, if they want to go with the same sex…I can't see anything wrong with it' (DO). Two other women expressed views that were tolerant or accepting, saying it was 'OK' (TY) or 'all right' (TM). The remaining thirteen held negative views, although only three of these were very strongly negative. The most commonly held opinions were that it was 'dirty', 'not nice' or 'wrong'. Clearly, most women had picked up commonly held prejudices against same-sex relationships, although it was not easy to see quite how these attitudes had developed. Only one woman actually knew a lesbian (her sister) and she had been influenced by her mother's reaction – 'my mum didn't like it very much…my mum thought it was terrible actually' (KN). None of the other women knew, or even knew of, any lesbian women. It is worth noting that these interviews took place before three of the major television soap operas (*EastEnders*, *Brookside* and *Emmerdale*) introduced lesbian characters. Television certainly can inform people with learning disabilities about sexual activities and relationships (see p.181) and one woman did say that the only gay person she had ever heard about was 'the man who used to be on *EastEnders*' (DY).

One of the most able women in the study recognised that lesbians and gay men experienced prejudice from others:

> MM: Do you think two women could have a good relationship?
>
> BN: They could, but not like what my boyfriend wants to do, get engaged and married.
>
> MM: No, they can't do those things, but that's not their fault, because there are laws …
>
> BN: It's not their fault. If a woman gets to like a woman she can't help it.
>
> MM: Do you think lesbians and gay men get treated properly by others or do some people give them a hard time?
>
> BN: I reckon some people give them a hard time, their friends might not want to know them any more if they find out.
>
> MM: What would you think if one of your friends told you she was a lesbian?
>
> AM: I might still go around with her but I might not. Because if I went around with her, *I'd* lose all my friends because they'd think I was a lesbian.
>
> MM: And you wouldn't want them to think that?
>
> AM: No, no.

Despite the fact that I didn't ask them to, a number of women made comparisons between heterosexual and same-sex relationships and expressed the view that same-sex relationships were very much 'second-best':

> It's nicer to have a boyfriend. (BN)

> If you're hard-up for a man, why go with a woman? (EY)

> It's better with a man and a woman, rather than two women or two men. (TM)

> It's all right for a man to play with a woman, but not two women. (TC)

The women were not speaking from their own experience here as they said that they had not had any sex with women and, moreover, they reported that their own experiences with men were largely unsatisfactory. They did not say, or imply, that anyone else had ever discussed lesbian sexuality with them. Nevertheless, they had formed their own opinions and these were largely negative.

Sexual dreams, thoughts and fantasies.

Sexual fantasy, in the commonly understood sense of term as an imagined scenario, was a difficult concept to explain to the women and, possibly due to this, I did not get the impression that any of them had sexual fantasies. It is important to note that I was not asking them to tell me what their fantasies were, merely whether they ever 'planned…imagined how sex might be' or 'look forward to it, thinking how you'd like it to be'. But no responses were forthcoming and I put this down to the abstract nature of the questioning and because it may have been too difficult or embarrassing a topic for the women to talk about. The difficulty of finding out whether people with learning disabilities have sexual fantasies has been noted elsewhere in the literature, albeit with a very different group – that is, male sexual offenders (O'Connor 1996). It is worth noting that the whole issue of fantasy and how it applies to people with learning disabilities more broadly is under-researched and, consequently, not well understood.

The more concrete (because they can be remembered as opposed to imagined) topic of dreams elicited a little more, but still limited, response. Two women each recounted a good dream that had been about sex but did not give the impression that this was something that had happened more than once. Three other women said that they sometimes did have dreams relating to sexuality and these varied from very good dreams (interestingly, two of these related to having a baby) to terrifying nightmares of being raped and stabbed. However, twelve women said that they never had dreams about sex. Two women pointed out to me, as though my question were somehow flawed, that they only dreamt about nice things: 'I dream good things, my parents and that, not sex' (FM); 'I only dream about interesting things, like going to the pictures, or seaside or on a day trip' (MH). These women seemed to be separating sex from other things which were sources of pleasure in their lives.

Ten of the twelve women who said they did not dream of sex when asleep also never thought about it when they were awake either and some were very clear about this, saying, in a firm tone, 'No, I don't think about it or dream about it or look forward to it at all' (JR).

One woman said she thought women didn't think about sex but that 'men thought about it all the time' (BN). She thought this because a male friend, who also lived in the same hospital for people with learning disabilities, had told her that 'all the men in the hospital think about sex and they wank themselves off' (BN). Another woman also said that she thought men thought and talked about sex more than women did and that this got on her nerves:

MM: Do you ever think about sex or dream about it?

KN: No, not really. I just get a bit worried when I hear about it – it unnerves me. I wish people would talk about something else.

MM: Who talks about it?

KN: G. [ex-boyfriend] used to talk about it and it used to get on my nerves, I used to say 'change the subject'.

MM: Do you ever hear women talking about sex?

KN: Not really.

Two women said that they did not dream about sex but sometimes did think about it when awake. For one woman this was having good thoughts remembering sex which had happened in the past; for the other it involved wishing for a better, more private environment where sex could be more than 'just five or ten minutes. People rush here because there are people around' (TM).

Overall, the women's perceptions of sex in their minds seemed somewhat sparse. Certainly, the wide variety of sexual fantasises and dreams which some women without learning disabilities report (Friday 1991) was absent. This contributes to the general impression the women give of sex being very much a physical experience and not one which has much, if any, of an emotional or psychological dimension. This will be discussed in more detail in the next chapter.

Someone to talk to

The women were asked whether there was anyone they felt they could talk to about sexual matters. Three indicated that there were a variety of avenues for this, including staff, mother, foster-mother, doctor. In addition, four women each said that there was one particular person they could talk to – for one woman this was her boyfriend (although she intimated that this did not, in fact, actually happen very often) and for the other three it was their female keyworker. A further three women answered the question hypothetically, saying that they felt they *could* talk to their female keyworker although, in fact, they never had. (They did, however, talk very readily to me). Three women said there was no one they could talk to.

However, of most concern (because it was the single most common response and because of what it says about staff in learning disability services) was the fact that seven women felt that although staff were theoretically available to them to discuss personal matters, in reality this was not the case:

> The staff don't always listen. (GJ)

> B. [male nurse] said to stop going on about my boyfriend. He said he didn't want to know about him. (MH)

> I talk to my named nurse about it sometimes, but she doesn't like talking about it. (DY)

As well as this was the fact that when staff did listen, their responses were sometimes simplistic and unhelpful – for example, to tell the women 'not to do it' (HC) or 'that I shouldn't go with the men' (EY). Also, two women were acutely aware of the power staff had, either to get information about their sexual lives or with regard to what they might do with it. One woman described how a woman doctor had questioned her:

> I told her about M. [boyfriend] and she said 'how many times has he had your body?' and I had to tell her, I couldn't cover it because she'd ring up and find out anyway. So you have to tell them the truth. (EY)

Another woman said that she did not want staff to know that she had sex with her boyfriend because 'they'll stop my money if I tell them' (TC). In fact, this was not true as the staff did know and they had not punished the

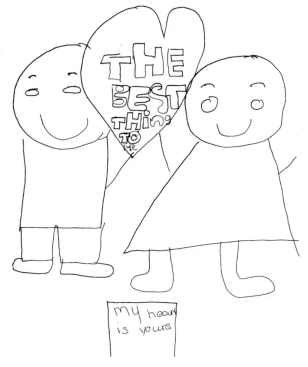

Figure 4.2

woman. But the point is that she *believed* it to be true and her fears were not unreasonable, taking the historical context into account. This woman had been in hospital for many years, quite possibly during the period when residents were, in fact, punished by staff for having relationships (Potts and Fido 1991).

With one or two exceptions who needed some prompting and persuasion, all the women had a lot they wanted to say about sex. Even though, at the outset at least, I was a stranger to most of them, they nevertheless had no problem filling several hours each with intimate discussions of their own sexual lives, as well as plenty of questions and discussion about sex more broadly. Given an opportunity to talk, explicit permission to do so and hearing me model open discussion of sexual matters, the women did not hold back. There was a sense of having opened the floodgates, although, sadly, I doubt that they remained open for very long. At the end of my work with every woman we identified who the most appropriate and approachable person was for her to talk to in the future. But I have little confidence that the opportunity would have been available on an ongoing basis. This is not necessarily a criticism of individual staff members, rather a reflection of services more broadly and will be discussed more fully in the section on recommendations (see p.240).

Knowledge of clitoris and orgasm

As so many of the women had responded negatively to the questions concerning their experience of sexual pleasure, further questions were asked concerning their knowledge of the part of their body most likely to produce sexual pleasure (i.e. clitoris) and the most overt or extreme manifestation of that pleasure (i.e. orgasm).

CLITORIS

Only two of the seventeen women seemed to know what the clitoris was. One woman said that she had heard about it from a diagram. This was a woman (TM) who had only borderline learning disabilities and who could, and did, read, so this is entirely possible. The other woman said that she knew about the clitoris because she had been taught about it on the child care course she was doing at college. Intrigued to know what would have been said about the clitoris on a child care course, I pursued this, only to realise she had confused the word 'clitoris' with the word 'uterus' and that, in fact, she knew nothing of the former.

The remaining fifteen women were also unaware of the existence of the clitoris – this means that they did not recognise the word (which I do not consider significant), nor did they seem to recognise it from my verbal attempts to describe it (usually in the following manner: 'it's a special part of women's privates, it's only small and feels a bit like a pea or something like that and it gives women good feelings when it's touched'), nor did they recognise it from a clear line drawing from my sex education package *Sex and the 3R's* (McCarthy and Thompson 1992).

In addition to the lack of awareness prior to my description, four women also expressed doubts as to whether they personally had a clitoris after I had explained to them what it was, for example:

I don't think I've got one. (MC).

I need to find out if I've got one. (EY).

I haven't got one of those. (TY).

ORGASM

Not surprisingly, in view of the above, none of the women seemed to have experienced orgasm. It should be noted that this is one of the most difficult areas to explore (Andron 1983) as, unlike other subjects, there are no pictures to show what an orgasm is. There are, however, sex education videos, including those made specifically for people with learning disabilities (such as *Piece By Piece* (West London Health Promotion Agency 1994) and *Feeling Sexy, Feeling Safe* (Family Planning Association of NSW 1993)) which show both women and men masturbating to orgasm. I did not use these in my research because they are extremely explicit (and, therefore, often cause embarrassment – to me as well as the other women) and I believe people should only be exposed to such material if there is a need to show them. In this situation I felt there was no need to introduce such explicit material. I was convinced, through my discussions generally, from the lack of knowledge of the clitoris and from the types of sexual activity they described having that they did not, in fact, experience orgasm. Interestingly, three of the most intellectually able women used slang terms, such as 'coming', and did initially report that they experienced this. However, on further questioning it transpired that they confused this with the experience of their vaginas becoming 'just all wet' (BN) or 'wet and ready for sex' (TM). I have noted elsewhere that this has been reported to me by more able women with learning disabilities (McCarthy 1996a).

For those women whose only or primary sexual contact was penetrative sex with men, it is easy to see how the clitoris could remain unexplored (and orgasm not experienced). Something that is not quite so easy to understand is the fact that the five women who said they did masturbate (or had done at some time) also did not know of their clitoris. This leads onto the question of precisely how the women masturbated. Hite's (1976) work indicates that women have a wide variety of techniques but that the clitoris plays a central role in almost all of them. Unfortunately, this was not an area I felt able to explore further with the women in this study. It was a subject that all the women appeared uncomfortable with to a greater or lesser degree and those women who said that they masturbated were, as I indicated earlier, very tentative in their admissions. I felt it would have been insensitive of me as a researcher, and inappropriate for me as a worker in the service, to push them into saying anything more about it than they were ready to.

MEN'S ORGASMS

Despite the absence of their own experience of orgasm, the women were quite well aware of the men's experiences of this. This reflects the situation of the much larger group of women with learning disabilities that I have worked with (McCarthy 1993). This is partly due to the physiological differences between men and women – that is, there is a visible outcome for men. I believe this is significant because the women often referred to what they had actually *seen* (most commonly referred to as 'the white stuff') and, sometimes, were unaware that there might be any particular feelings associated with this for men. However, it is primarily due to the fact that the men *were* having orgasms.

Two of the seventeen women did not appear to understand my questions related to this and a further two understood but were not sure whether the men they had sex with experienced orgasm or not. The remaining thirteen women, however, were quite clear that this happened regularly with their partners:

MM: What happens to a man's body when he has sex?

GJ: Willy goes up.

MM: Yes, anything else?

GJ: Sperm.

MM: Yes and when that sperm comes out, that gives the man good feelings.

GJ: That's what happens to S. [boyfriend], he gets worked up and I get a bit scared.

That white stuff always comes out. (TY)

The semen, jelly stuff, white comes out. (TM)

GN: They can give you a baby.

MM: That's right, because something comes out of the penis, doesn't it?

GN: Bank…the white stuff.

MM: It's called sperm.

GN: Sperm…I told you, sperm bank.

Although I did not specifically explore this with anyone, four women clearly explained that they had an active role to play in helping men to achieve orgasm, for example:

> M. gets me to rub his willy and he's always saying 'I'm coming'. (MC)

> But if you've got your time of the month and they want it, all you can do for them is wank them off. (EY)

> Most men like you to play with their cock and that helps them to come. (BN)

The last woman also went on to describe how men liked to ejaculate over women's bodies: 'They prefer to come over the woman than over themselves, because they enjoy it more' (BN). The above information, combined with the fact that none of the women's partners felt it was their role to reciprocate and give sexual pleasure to the women, consolidates the picture that is starting to form of the women providing a sexual service to the men.

Types of sexual activity

One woman declined to give details, therefore the following information concerns sixteen women. Responses were divided down the middle with eight women experiencing only penetrative sex and eight women who had a variety of sexual experiences, within which penetration played a central role. Of those who only experienced penetrative sex, four had had both vaginal and anal intercourse and four vaginal intercourse only. Three of the eight said that this might be occasionally accompanied by kissing but not always. For the rest of the sixteen, kissing was not mentioned, although this may possibly be due to the fact that at this point I was specifically asking about sex and kissing may not be defined as 'sex'. However, I did have sex education pictures available to help the women describe their experiences and these did contain images of women and men kissing.

Eight women had had a variety of sexual experiences – three women had had men stimulating them by hand to achieve lubrication (see below); for the remaining five, the 'variety' was, in fact, the woman stimulating the man's penis by hand.

The women's responses to questions and pictures (where these were used) of oral sex were very interesting. Only two women had ever experienced a man giving them oral sex and each of these had only experienced it once. Neither had found it a particularly positive experience – one because she thought it was disgusting and it had tickled her so much she kept moving around; the other didn't say how *she* had felt about it, only that the man reported feeling sick afterwards and her conclusion was that 'he shouldn't have done it' (EY). In total, nine women spoke in very strong and negative terms about giving oral sex to a man:

> I don't like this one at all, it's a horrible taste. (MC)

> I don't mind normal sex and kissing and cuddling, but I don't like giving them blow-jobs. (BN)

> That's a thing I don't like, it makes me feel sick. (EY)

Of the remaining seven, five had no experience of it, one did not say anything about it and one woman said she enjoyed it. This last woman is, in fact, the only woman with learning disabilities from the seventy or so I have worked with who has spoken of this particular activity in positive terms. The widespread dislike and strength of feeling about this sexual activity has been noted elsewhere in my work (McCarthy 1993, 1994) and I had hoped to use this research to try to understand this phenomenon more fully. Although this research does confirm the overwhelmingly negative feelings associated with this activity, unfortunately, I was not able to discover quite *why* so many women with learning disabilities dislike it so much more than other sexual activities. Certainly, it is the case that, like others, some women with learning disabilities have picked up negative associations with this sexual activity that are not based on their own experience. Indeed, three of the nine who expressed the strongest feelings about it said they had never experienced it and had no intention of doing so, believing that it was 'disgusting' (the most commonly used word to describe it by all the women; 'filthy' and 'vulgar' being other terms). The other six women said that they had experienced the activity but it was clear that it was not as common as penetrative sex and that the women did, where possible, refuse men's requests for this. Of the six who had experienced it and disliked it, three specified that it was the taste they disliked and another mentioned feeling sick. For another woman it was also the physical side of the experience she disliked: 'It makes my jaw ache…it's uncomfortable' (TM). One woman believed that she could become pregnant from oral sex:

> EY: The stuff goes in your mouth.

> MM: Do you mind that?

> EY: It can make you sick, make you pregnant.

> MM: No, not that way.

EY: Can't you? How do you know?

MM: You can only get pregnant if the sperm goes in your vagina.

EY: You can't get pregnant if it goes in your mouth? Are you sure?

MM: Positive.

EY: Well you've taught me something there.[1]

As well as the physical side of things, two women mentioned the interaction with men which made them annoyed or uncomfortable – for example, 'Lots of them ask you to do this. They think it's bloody great. They get the thrill because they're going to have it in her mouth' (MC). Another woman said that the men *said* they would take their penis out of her mouth before they ejaculated but, in fact, did not.

It is clear from all the women in this study, and, indeed, the much larger group of women I have worked with, that most of their sexual activity focuses on stimulation of the penis.

The following diagram shows the most and least common sexual activities as reported by the women (both those in this study and the bigger group I have worked with).

Most Common

Penetrative sex
(always vaginal, often anal)
↕
Woman touching man's genitals
↕
Oral sex from woman to man
↕
Man touching woman's genitals
↕
Oral sex from man to woman

Least Common

[1]   This woman was 55 years old, had been sexually active with men for many years and had had two children.

Few women experienced the same kinds of genital stimulation as the men and other sensitive parts of their bodies were largely ignored. Rather surprisingly, given that they are both sexual and sexualised body parts, breasts were only mentioned twice throughout all the interviews – one woman saying that, sometimes, men liked to ejaculate over hers and another woman complaining that men had squeezed her breasts too hard and hurt her.

Experiencing physical pain from sexual activity[2]

Two fairly simple questions were asked on whether pain was experienced during sex and what the women's responses were to this. It turned out to be a very fruitful area of discussion with the women not only providing me with their own experiences and responses but also with a wealth of information about the men's responses too.

Answers to the question whether sex ever hurt them came in three categories: no; yes, sometimes; and a more definite yes (meaning the woman indicated it either always happened and/or the pain was severe). Three women said that sex did not hurt them, although one of these distinguished between the times it had hurt – that is, when she had been raped and the times it did not hurt – that is, her consenting sex with her boyfriend. Eight women said that sex sometimes hurt them and the remaining six women said that it definitely or always hurt them. Thus it is the case that the significant majority of women (fourteen of seventeen) in this sample experience sex as painful on more than a one-off or occasional basis. This is also true for the very many of the other women with learning disabilities I have worked with. For all the women, it was penetrative sexual intercourse which caused the pain – no other sexual activity was mentioned in this context. Pain arising from anal intercourse only was mentioned by two women, with a further seven specifying that it was both anal and vaginal intercourse which caused pain. Five women only mentioned vaginal intercourse as painful and indicated that they had no experience of anal intercourse. This means that all of the women who did experience anal intercourse experienced it as painful.

Some of the women believed that sex was meant to hurt (see also Andron and Ventura 1987), although whether they had been told this or deduced it from their own experience is not known:

2   For the possible experience of emotional or psychological distress caused by sex, see p.198 on how sex makes the women feel about themselves.

MM: Is sex supposed to hurt or not?

MC: I don't think it hurts men but it is supposed to hurt a woman. I don't know if that's right or not.

MM: Is sex supposed to hurt women? Is it how it's meant to be?

TC: Yes it's meant to hurt.

MM: Is it meant to hurt men as well?

TC: Just women.

MM: Why is it meant to hurt women?

TC: I don't know why.

However, as neither vaginal nor anal intercourse are necessarily painful experiences, I asked the women about natural and artificial lubrication. Two women (both having sex with men with learning disabilities in hospitals) said that, occasionally, the men produced *Vaseline* and used this for lubrication for anal sex. Both said that the men refused to put it on their penises and, instead, applied it to the women's body, which, perhaps, accounted for the fact that it was largely ineffective in reducing the pain. (Although she did not mention it at the time of this interview, I knew from work a few years previously that another woman's boyfriend (also a man with learning disabilities in hospital) had used shampoo for the same purpose and to the same (lack of) effect.) One of the women who had said that one partner had used lubrication clearly saw this as the man's responsibility and blamed another partner for not having done so:

> Well why didn't M. think of that then when he had me the back way? He must be stupid. (EY)

Three other women (all the most intellectually able, two of whom were referring to sex with men without learning disabilities) indicated that there was, sometimes, natural vaginal lubrication, achieved by the men briefly stimulating the women with their hand. All three women specifically said that this sexual activity was for the purpose of achieving lubrication for penetration and not part of sex for its own sake. As one woman poignantly said, 'Men do this to warn women of what is coming next, they want sex' (MC). Two of these three women framed the achieving of vaginal lubrication as something which made intercourse easier for men, as the conversation with BN shows:

BN: [hesitantly] Sometimes they like to make you wet before they put it in you, 'cos they find it easier. They finger you, to make it easier for them to get it in.

MM: But doesn't it make it more comfortable for *you* too, if you're wet?

BN: I don't mind. If you're dry, they have to poke you about, to find the hole, to get it up…so it's better for them if you're wet.

MM: Isn't it better for *you* as well as them?

BN: I don't mind.

For the remaining twelve women, there was no lubrication of vagina or anus prior to penetration, hence the frequency with which pain was experienced.

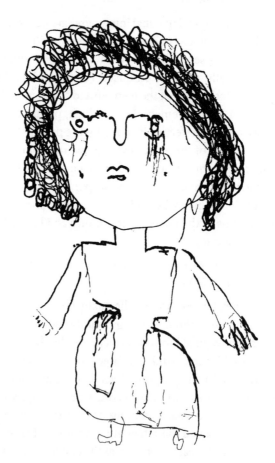

Figure 4.3

Of the fourteen women who experienced physical pain during sex, none was able to resolve the situation by informing her partner that it hurt and negotiating a more mutually comfortable activity. In terms of causing the pain to cease, the best that could happen was that two women were able to complain sufficiently to bring about the end of that particular sexual encounter. Neither woman indicated that this happened every time sex hurt but, rather, occasionally. For the other twelve women (and, sometimes, for the above two women as well) it was a case of them feeling that they had to put up with it. By this I do not mean to imply that they felt it was 'a woman's lot' to suffer pain in silence (although, as stated above, three women did believe that sex was supposed to hurt women and not men). Rather, nine of the women had, in fact, attempted to tell the men they had sex with that they were being hurt and had got anything from a less than satisfactory to a downright punitive response from the men concerned:

> They just carry on. (GJ)

> He gets a bit upset, in a bad mood. (GN)

> I tell them to go away, they *won't* go away, they *keep* on doing it. (TD)

MM: So what do you do when it still hurts?

MC: There's not a lot you can do.

MM: So what *do* you do?

MC: Nothing.

MM: Do you ever say that it hurts or say 'ouch'?

MC: I cry.

MM: Do you cry while they're doing it or after it's finished?

MC: Whilst they're doing it because it's very, very painful.

MM: And what do they do when you cry?

MC: Nothing, they just carry on. They say 'what's the matter with you, cry-baby.' They tell you to shut up and go rougher.

MM: What would you like them to do?

MC: I'd like them to stop there and then, but they don't.

A possible reason why some men with learning disabilities may not respond more appropriately is that they find it difficult to comprehend that *their* experience is not *the* experience. In other words, as a person with learning disabilities, they may well have difficulty with abstract thinking and are unable to imagine that another person would be experiencing things differently from themselves. One indication of this was given by a woman who said: 'I told him it was hurting but he just said "it don't hurt"' (KS). In other words, because it was not hurting him, it was not hurting. However, this by no means explains the behaviour of all the men – some had no learning disability at all and others only mild learning disabilities, therefore they should not have had any particular difficulty in comprehending the other person's experience. Moreover, sex education work with men with learning disabilities has shown that it is, in fact, quite common for the men to be indifferent to their partner's quality of experience (Gardiner, Kelly and Wilkinson 1996).

Five women specifically said that it was their fear of the men's adverse, often violent, reaction which prevented them from trying to speak out:

> MM: What do you think he'd do?
>
> MC: Beat me up…He's a great bloody tall bleeder and most of the girls here are frightened of him. He's bigger than I am, I'm not used to giants. [The man in question was approximately 6' 4", well built and nearly everyone, including staff, was afraid of him.]

> If I was to tell a man to stop, he might do the opposite. (FM) [This woman had been raped by a fellow pupil at a residential school.]

> MM: So you can't tell him?
>
> TC: No, because he doesn't like it, he goes for me if I tell him. [This woman's boyfriend was known to, in her own words, 'thump' her for various reasons.]

In light of the above, I think it is important to challenge the view that women with learning disabilities are essentially passive and unassertive when it comes to sex with men – a view which comes as much from my own previous work as other people's. Rather, a more rounded view is that, on occasions at least, women with learning disabilities, like many others in difficult situations, make considered decisions about their personal safety. Sometimes, they have to trade off one kind of physical pain in order to avoid another.

Sex during menstruation

Throughout the course of my sexuality work generally with women with learning disabilities, a number of women had said that having a period was given, and largely received, by men as a 'legitimate' reason for refusing sex (this is also common amongst heterosexuals in the general population; see Holland *et al.* 1998). However, quite how the women managed to impart this information to men is not clear, as many women in this study said that they did not like to talk about this with men as it was too embarrassing:

> I can't tell them when I'm on the other way. (TC)

> I don't like telling my period to him. (KS)

The women were asked how they felt about having sex during a period. All disapproved, including the one woman who had done it on occasions. Most had fairly pragmatic reasons for this, with five citing the mess that would be caused and two more citing period pains or pre-menstrual tension as reasons why they would not have sex at this time. In addition, most also felt it was inherently wrong, not allowed, embarrassing, disgusting to have sex during a period:

> I wouldn't do that because if you're having ladies' troubles and there was blood coming out, it would be disgusting. (FM)

> HC: Not when you've got your period. I don't do it when I've got my period.
>
> MM: Why is that?
>
> HC: You mustn't.
>
> MM: Who said you mustn't?
>
> HC: You mustn't do it.

Four also felt there could be physiological consequences, with two suggesting some kind of bodily damage (see also Andron 1983) and two suggesting an increased risk of pregnancy.

Preferred sexual activities

The women were asked which, of the sexual activities they engaged in, they liked most or least. Three women did not know or did not say and two said they did not like anything. For the rest, the picture was more complex, with some women giving first and second choices for what they liked best and first and second choices for what they liked least. Others simply stated one thing they liked most. The overall picture which emerges is that just kissing and cuddling was preferred by one-third of the women:

> I didn't mind him giving me a kiss at all...it's just the sex thing he did to me...I didn't like that. (JR)

FM: I like kissing.

MM: Good, anything else?

FM: I don't like the part where he gets on top of you.

A further six women named vaginal intercourse as their preferred activity – two of these women did not have any other sexual activities and the other four were clearly comparing it to anal intercourse, which they all named as least preferred activity. Indeed, it was difficult to get a sense of what, if anything, was preferred in its own right and the way the questions were worded – that is, 'what do you like doing best/least?' – did lead people to rate activities against each other.

Notwithstanding the above, anal intercourse was definitely rated negatively by all – many named it as the least favoured and no one named it as their best activity. Some women expressed their views about it in strong terms and this seemed to be due to the pain it caused:

> Not many people like it in the anus, men do but not women. It hurts, it's dreadful, very very painful and not a nice one. If you're out with a fella and they demand point blank range that they give it up the bum and you don't want them to do so and they keep on pestering you, so you don't know whether to say yes or no and it bloody hurts... (MC)

Strong feelings were also expressed regarding the women giving oral sex to men, with many women naming it as a least favoured activity. However, nobody mentioned that this was painful. It was disliked for other reasons, few of which were specific (see p.140 above for general discussion). Only one woman said that oral sex on a man was the thing she liked to do best. This woman was the one who was very positive about all her sexual experiences. (Lest it be thought she was someone who said she liked everything, it should be noted that she was, in fact, well able to say when she did not like something, having complained about aspects of the service she received, for example.)

The women's perceptions of men's preferred sexual activities

Seven women either did not know or did not say which sexual activities they thought men preferred. Of the remaining ten, seven believed that men preferred penetrative sex (four said vaginal, two said anal and one said men liked

both equally). Two women said that they thought kissing was the least preferred activity for men. Three women said that there was nothing that men
did not like sexually. Two of them expressed very definite views on this:

MM: What do you think men like doing least?

BN: That's a hard one for *men*, they like everything. They wouldn't refuse
a thing, the men.

They just see a woman and jump on her and it's bad. Men haven't got
much good taste, if you know what I mean. (MH)

They're not bloody bothered. They like it all. The only thing they don't
like is those condoms. (MC)

This last woman had a very low opinion of men's sexual conduct generally:

Well any man, no matter on the street, in hospital, married or unmarried,
there is *no* and I tell you this and you're wrong if you say there is, there is
no fucking decent fellas, not anywhere in the world today, because they
just pounce on you in the middle of nowhere and just start on you for sex.
There's a lot of fucking savages nowadays. (MC)

This low opinion was partly based on her own experience: during the time I
was interviewing her and she made the above statement, she was sexually
assaulted by a man with learning disabilities in the hospital who *had* literally
pounced on her and left her with extensive facial bruising. However, she also
formed her views from her wider knowledge of men's sexual behaviour and
sexual attacks, which she gleaned from the media, and she made even stron-
ger statements about men whose behaviour she differentiated as being more
extreme than the others. After news reports of a serious sexual assault on a
seven-year-old girl which took place during the time I was interviewing her,
she said:

There are some bastard cunts of men in this England who attack young
kids. No matter where they lurk, these men, they've always got a crazed
killing sensation in their heads. How honestly does he think he's going
to fucking get away with it? I bet he will. They're crazy, men like that.
(MC)

Although her language is a little lurid, the strength of her feeling of outrage
about the sexual assaults that were taking place was very real. However, I
think she was fairly exceptional and none of the other women I spoke to gave

me any reason to believe that they based their opinions on anything other than their own personal experiences.

Fear associated with sex

The women were asked if there was anything about sex which frightened them. Three said that there was not and another three said that it had been scary at first – that is, when they were younger – but that had passed as it had become a more familiar experience. Two women said that everything about sex was frightening – one was a young woman who had relatively recently started her first sexual relationship. The other woman who found everything about sex frightening put this down to 'thinking about my dad, about getting pregnant and stuff. But I hope I'll get over it and won't be frightened about getting pregnant' (KN). This woman had been raped by her father and had given birth to his child, so it is not surprising that both elements of this experience still loomed large in her mind. However, what does not come across in her own words is any sense of time-scale: she was, in fact 'still hoping to get over it' some 31 years later and her fears of pregnancy had not diminished despite being 48 and having the Depo-Provera injection.

Nine other women said that there were things about sex which frightened them. Interestingly, despite the fact that the location for sex was often very unsatisfactory (see below), only one woman mentioned anything to do with the time or place for sex, saying it was scary to do it in the dark. For all the others it was something about the sexual interaction itself which sometimes frightened them: for a few it was certain kinds of sexual activity (vaginal intercourse, having the vagina touched, oral sex on a man); for others it was a fear of potential sexual violence 'if a man forces himself on you, rape' (EY); for others it was a fear of physical violence that might take place alongside sex 'I'm frightened he might hit me in the mouth, he's a bully' (GJ).

Payment for sex

From my wider experience of sexuality work with women with learning disabilities, many women in hospitals had told me that they were given small sums of money or cigarettes (occasionally drinks and sweets) by men for sex. This was understood by both the women and men as payment. Consequently, all the women in this study were asked if they received payment and what they thought about the issue. The findings were striking, with there being a clear split in responses depending on whether the women were living in a hospital or community setting. All the eight women living in hospitals had received payment; none of the seven community-based women had. Of the two women who usually lived in the community but who were in hospital at the time of being interviewed, one was being given money by her boyfriend (a long-term hospital resident) and the other was not (her boyfriend was newly arrived in the hospital for the first time himself). These findings clearly confirm earlier assertions of mine that the exchange of sex for money is an integral part of the institutional subculture (McCarthy 1993). That it is to do with the nature of the institutional context and not the nature of the people placed there is clearly demonstrated by the fact that it is not a prevalent practice in community learning disability services. Furthermore, the attitudes towards accepting payment differed depending on where the women lived. The hospital-based women not only accepted but *expected* money, believing that this was the right thing and that it was not fair if men did not pay them. The conversation with EY illustrates this:

> EY: I have been with some men who were no good and didn't give me a penny. What would you do if you were going with a man who had a lot of money and never gave you anything?

> MM: I wouldn't expect him to give me money.

> EY: But if you'd been giving him things?

> MM: If I gave him presents and things like that, then yes, I would expect him to give me presents too sometimes, but not money.

In my response to the woman here I am attempting to distinguish between reciprocal gift-giving between partners and payment of one by the other.

In contrast to those in hospital, the community-based women all expressed the view that it was wrong to exchange sex for money:

> I think it's wrong, you shouldn't be having sex if you're charging people, like prostitutes, tarts, it's disgusting. (DY)

> Men paying girls is the wrong thing to do. (LT)

Interestingly, this last woman was the only one to comment on the men's behaviour – all the other women, whether they approved or not, spoke of women accepting payment, not of men offering it. This focus on the woman's role in the exchange is a reflection of society's traditional view of prostitution where the women are stigmatised and criminalised rather than their male clients. Moreover, in terms of attempting to understand the issue, looking only at reasons why women accept money and not at why men offer it is to miss at least half the point (Jeffreys 1985). However, in recent years there have been some, albeit isolated, examples of initiatives which seek to seek to redress this imbalance and which work from an explicitly feminist perspective in focusing on men's role in purchasing sexual services (see, for example, Monto 1998).

The women with learning disabilities in this study were fully aware that men paid women and not the other way around. My questions as to whether women ever did, or should, pay men for sex was met with anything from a complete lack of understanding of the concept, to an incredulous laugh, to me being patronised for seeming to ask such a stupid question: 'Well I'll give you a few basic tips there…' (MC). The fact that the subculture of the institution largely reflects the exchange of sex for money in the outside world should come as no surprise and, consequently, might be viewed by some as 'natural' and of little concern. However, as paying can bring with it the power to control what happens in the encounter, it clearly should be viewed with concern, especially when those who are paying and, therefore, 'calling the shots' are already advantaged by gender and, often, by a greater intellectual ability and physical size. However, although it would be easy to view the women as simply being exploited by men in these exchanges, I think this would be overly simplistic. As sexual pleasure was largely or entirely missing for the women, the women themselves saw taking money as a way of getting something from the encounters. This was expressed by one woman in her usual vivid manner: 'Men see us a bloody garbage user, use us to do what they want and turn their backs. So basically if they have got any money in their pockets to pay for having a woman and doing what they want, then, yes, fucking charge them' (MC).

Receiving something from the encounter went some way, in some women's minds, to equalising the situation somewhat. Indeed, a number of women described how men made false promises regarding payment and this was very much resented. I have written elsewhere how some women describe this payment as having been 'earned' by them (McCarthy 1993):

> He doesn't usually give the things he's promised. Sometimes but not usually. (MC)

> He shows me £10 first, but he doesn't give it to me afterwards. (GJ)

In the course of my broader sex education work I was referred a number of women who had had sex for money, but I never tried merely to dissuade them from accepting such reward. This is because it is hard to justify why the men should receive what was, in fact, a servicing of their sexual needs for nothing.

Rather, I worked with the women more broadly to attempt to increase what they got from their sexual encounters. Although this would appear to be a clash of values between myself and other staff within the services, it never proved difficult to overcome. Most staff readily took on board the fact that it would be very difficult to try to dissuade a few individuals from doing something that many other people in their social milieu were doing and which was widely accepted or viewed as inevitable.

Where sex took place

Once again, clear differences emerged depending on whether the women were in hospital or community settings. All seven women in the community said that they had sex at home in the bedroom, usually theirs but occasionally the man's. The importance of staff being clear to women that they could use their own bedrooms for sex if they wanted to was starkly illustrated by two women who lived in the same service (a small group home) yet who had formed quite different views of what was allowed. One believed she could not have that kind of privacy at home:

> Here? [incredulous tone] Can't do it here, it's rented from [name of organisation]. I go around his house. (LT)

Whereas her fellow resident said:

> Yes, because in my room is my own private place, no one else is allowed to come and annoy us or anything, the door is locked. (DO)

One community-based woman who did have privacy available also had had sex in a semi-private place in her day centre. In contrast, all the hospital-based women (including the two normally in the community) conducted their sexual lives outdoors or in semi-private places indoors, such as back staircases or unused rooms. It is important to note that some of these women did have their own bedrooms – one chose not to have her boyfriend in her room (although staff had explicitly said she could) because she valued it as her own private space and she did not want him there. Mostly, however, there were rules against the women taking men into their rooms, sometimes onto the ward itself. Whilst these rules seem, and often are, unreasonable infringements on people's freedom, it is not always as simple an issue as it may seem at face value. For instance, two of the women in this study were on wards which were home to several vulnerable women. Both had boyfriends who were convicted sex offenders and staff prevented the men from coming onto the wards, feeling that they were acting wisely to safeguard their vulnerable clients.

Some of the hospital-based women expressed concern about their lack of privacy:

> MM: Would you like to have a more private place for sex?
>
> EY: If it was more private, you could have sex without anybody seeing you and opening their mouth about you.

> Yes I would, where no one else can see what I'm doing. I don't like patients seeing me, they've got no right to see me. (TC)

> It would be better, there'd be no people looking over the fence or coming around. (TM)

The outdoor settings in hospitals were the backs of buildings (including a disused mortuary), bushes and secluded areas. In addition, two of the four hospitals included in this study had places (a shed and a caravan) which were well known and well used by many different residents to have sex in – indeed, old mattresses had been placed in them for that purpose (though by whom I do not know). Although I did not personally see the shed, many women described it as 'not very nice'. If it was anything like the caravan, this is a serious understatement. About a year after the sex education team began its work, a woman with learning disabilities offered to show me the caravan she and many others had sex in. I could not believe what I was seeing and, because I was with her, I struggled to control my emotions and cut the visit short. I returned later that day with my male colleague and we were both stunned into silence and nearly moved to tears by the sight: it was a wreck, littered with broken glass, filth (including excrement of some kind) and rubbish. We took photos of it as we hoped that in the long term we might be able to persuade the hospital management to substantially improve the conditions. As a short-term measure, we went out and bought lots of cleaning materials, stayed behind after work and scrubbed the place from top to bottom, put in clean sheets, etc.

This is an extreme example (I hope) and, as I have indicated above, most hospital residents had sex round the backs of buildings, in the bushes, etc. However, I have told the story of the caravan because it *was* regularly used as a location for sex and because, despite its horrors, it was chosen, presumably, because it offered at least some protection from the elements and some degree of privacy. Although many women and men spoke of using the caravan, none complained of the condition of it and I think this indicates something of the psychological and emotional 'blocking' that some people with learning disabilities would need to employ when they are forced to conduct their sexual relations in circumstances other people would not tolerate. (As a postscript to the caravan story, I should add that when confronted with the evidence of the state of the caravan, the hospital managers did not seek to improve it but had it removed from the site).

Whether clothing was removed during sex

Two women did not answer these questions. Of the remaining fifteen, four regularly experienced sex with no clothes on. Three of these were women who had sex in bed with men who were also undressed. The fourth was in the outdoor semi-private places described above. The other eleven women mostly or always had sex with their clothes on, removing only what was necessary for sex to take place. The men did not get undressed either. Three of these women would occasionally get fully undressed – all said that this was at the men's request or insistence and that the men did not reciprocate, despite the fact that the women wanted them to. Two women specifically recognised this as 'not fair' and one just said that she did not like it:

> …Not usually naked, only sometimes. In winter I don't take my clothes off. In summer I do sometimes, but the men don't. I have asked them to, but they say no. It's not fair. (MC)

> MH: He didn't like taking his trousers off.

> MM: Why was that?

> MH: He told me to take all my clothes off. He used to take his trousers down but keep his shirt and tie on.

> MM: So why did he get you to take all your clothes off?

> MH: That's the way he used to do it.

> MM: Do you think that was fair?

> MH: I didn't like the idea of it, it got a bit cold.

Decision making and sexual activity

The women were asked who made the decisions whether to have sex, where and how. Five women said that these decisions got made by either or both partners, although one of them said that men might consult women but did not always and went on to describe what was essentially a rape scenario. One woman said that she made the decisions – this seemed accurate as far as the decision whether to have sex was concerned but contradicted what she had previously said about the type of sexual activity she had. On the one hand, she was saying that it was up to her what sexual activity she had with her partner but, on the other hand, she said that she did not like the sex that took place and wanted something else. Whilst it is possible that she was actively choosing sex she did not like (as a form of self-punishment, for example) I have no reason to think so and assume, perhaps, that there was something about the questions which confused her.

Eleven women said that it was the men who made the decisions about sex, although a few indicated that this was not always a conscious process. For example, one said that she and her boyfriend only ever had vaginal intercourse, therefore there was nothing to decide regarding the type of sex. Another women said that she always had sex with an ex-hospital resident when he came back to visit his girlfriend (not her). She implied that this was their routine and it did not take much thinking about.

Three of the eleven women specifically said that they would like to have more say in what went on:

MM: Who decides what kind of sex you have?

EY: The man does, the man, but the woman should tell him.

MM: What happens with you?

EY: I should decide and he should decide.

MM: That's what should happen, but what does happen?

EY: The man decides.

MM: Do you think it's OK that men make all the decisions?

EY: [very definitely] No I don't, not all the time.

MM: Would you like to make more decisions about sex?

EY: Yes, I'd want the man to agree with me.

I think the women should get more of a choice to say if they want it or not. I think it's more cruel to make girls have sex when they don't want it, when they're not ready to. (LT)

One woman gave me an example of how she did sometimes take control by resisting what the men wanted from her: 'When they say to me have it up the anus, I say "you fucking piss off" and I run away, 'cos it's painful up the bum' (TD).

As well as being asked who made the decision to have sex in the first place, the women were asked who, if anyone, decided when or how each sexual encounter was going to end. Five women did not respond to this question at all, which was unusual, and those who did answer often had a puzzled or confused look on their face. I got the impression that they thought I was a bit stupid, asking such a question when the answer was so obvious. Nine women said that sex ended when the man had his orgasm. Once again, it was clear from what the women said that this was not a conscious decision on anyone's part but just the way things were – that is, that *was* how sex ended:

> MM: Who decides when sex has finished?
>
> GJ: I don't know what you mean.
>
> MM: Well, how do you know when sex has finished, when to stop?
>
> GJ: It finishes when the sperm comes out.

> MM: Does sex ever carry on after the man's sperm has come out?
>
> DO: No, that's when it's finished.

> MM: How do you know when sex is over?
>
> KN: The fella does, don't he?
>
> MM: How do they know?
>
> KN: When his thrill's over, it finished.

However, two women said that sex ended in other ways: for one, it was when the time came for her to go back to her ward for her next meal; for the other, it was when she got fed up with it, indicating that she did have some control over matters.

Women taking the initiative

The women were asked if they ever had, or ever would, ask (in words or actions) a man to have sex with them. Three did not respond. Three said that it would be unusual but that they possibly would or, occasionally, had. One woman distinguished between her long-term boyfriend and other more casual partners: 'I couldn't, I'd be embarrassed. I'd tell D. but not other men, I know my boyfriend for a long time' (GN). One woman clearly recognised when she felt attracted to a man and said that she would take the initiative 'if I took a liking to someone and I wanted a bit of romance' (EY). Another woman, by asking a man with learning disabilities into her bed, did seem to be asking for sex (and that was certainly what happened). But, at other points in the interview, she said clearly that she wanted kissing and cuddling, not the penetrative sex which took place. Unlike the above woman, this woman was not able to identify (or at any rate share with me) that it was her attraction to a particular man and/or feelings of sexual arousal that prompted her to ask the man into her bed. In fact, she said that she did not know why she did it.

The remaining ten women all said that they would never ask a man for sex. These included two women who had reputations (amongst staff and other residents in hospital) for having sex with a number of men for money or cigarettes. It was reported by staff that the women initiated at least some of these exchanges but whether they had actually observed this or just imagined it would be the case is not clear. The women themselves, whilst they readily admitted taking money and cigarettes for sex, said that they did not ask the men but were asked by them.

Choosing a partner

As well as enquiring into who took the initiative with regards to sexual activity, the women were also asked who initiated the relationships they had – for example, who approached whom, who asked the other to be their boyfriend/girlfriend. One woman did not have a relationship or arrangement with anybody and two others did not respond. Eleven women said that men generally or always chose them and asked them out. Most did not express any view on this. Again, it was just the way things were. Two women, however, did express the view (one very strongly) that this was the proper order of things, that it was men's role to do this, not women's. Another woman took a slightly different view, expressing (in her tone of voice as well as her words) her dissatisfaction:

> MM: Do you choose the men you go out with or do they choose you?
>
> MC: They choose me.
>
> MM: Why is it that way around?
>
> MC: I don't really have a lot of choice.

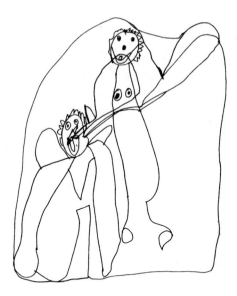

Figure 4.4 'He's stunned she's after him – she made the first move'

> MM: Why do you think that is, that they always choose you and you
> don't get to choose them?
>
> MC: That's just the way they work.

Another woman, in describing a typical sexual encounter, gave a very elo-
quent and poignant account of what could be a one-off sexual encounter or
could develop into an ongoing relationship:

> A man looks at you, then if he likes you, he says he wants to go with you
> and do something with you. Then he says 'lay down, I want to interfere
> with you', or 'I want your body', because he likes you. Then he lays down
> on top of you, puts his arms around you and kisses you, then he puts his
> thing up you, then he gets off you and says he'll see you again and thank
> you and all that, for giving me your body and maybe he says he loves you,
> then he says he gotta to go now. (EY)

One woman said that it was usually men who approached her but that she
had asked her current boyfriend out.

Two other women said that it could happen either way around – one of
these was a woman who was actively, and very inappropriately, pursuing a
male doctor in the hospital, trying to form a relationship with him.

Reasons to have sex

This proved a difficult thing for many women to think about. Some of the intellectually most able women commented on how difficult a question it was, something they would have to think about. After time for discussion and thought, in fact, three women (not the most able) could not give any reasons why they had sex. The fourteen other women did all say what their reasons were. These varied greatly and some women had only one reason whilst others had several. One or two women said that they had different reasons with different men – that is, it depended on the circumstances:

> MC: Mainly if I know they're really wealthy and they say 'can I have sex with you?' I say 'well what've you got to produce then?'
>
> MM: So is one of the reasons you have sex with men for the money?
>
> MC: Yes and for cigarettes.
>
> MM: Any other reasons?
>
> MC: Well with P. I did it for him more or less because I was in love with him and I've never felt that way about anyone else.

The single most common reason given (by six women) was loving or liking the men they had sex with. Another women did not use the words 'love' or 'like' but said that she did it because she wanted to marry her boyfriend in the future, which I took to be in the same category of responses. Three women said that they had sex because they liked it and another said that having sex made her feel 'more in control of my own life. If I don't want it, I can say no. If I do want it, I just keep going along with it' (DO).

Four women said that one, or only, reason for having sex was getting money or cigarettes. Another three said that *they* did not have any reasons and implied that they did not actively engage in sex, rather it was *done to them* by men. Their lack of active involvement in sex was graphically illustrated by an incident involving one woman (GJ), which was reported to me by a member of staff and later confirmed by the woman herself as accurate and typical: the staff member walked in on the woman having sex with her regular partner (an ex-hospital resident who came to visit his girlfriend, a different woman) in a staff rest room. The woman was leaning over a table, being penetrated from behind. She was eating a packet of crisps and appeared to be not much interested or 'involved' in what was happening. This emotional or psychological 'disengagement' from the physical activity was (although by no means universal for the women in this study) not uncommon. The women who reported having sex for money also seemed to distance themselves emotionally from what happened, as did those who had sex because they felt they had to for fear of men's reactions if they did not. Gavey's (1992) research also concluded that 'when sex is engaged in for pragmatic reasons, it can take on specific meaning as something which is mundane, an ordinary physical activity' (p.344.) One woman said several times throughout the interview that she engaged in sex which she neither liked nor wanted as a way of placating men – 'to shut them up' and 'to keep the peace' (KN).

Although having a baby was mentioned by a few women at different points in the interviews, only one mentioned it in the context of it being a reason to have sex. This woman mentioned it as the fifth of her six reasons and, interestingly, hesitated before she told me, prefacing it with the remark 'you might think it's disgusting if I told you' (EY). The fact that she thought I would be disgusted if she told me she had sex because she wanted a baby, but not that she took money for sex, is an indication of the messages she had been given about what was, and was not, acceptable for someone like her. Sadly for her, there was no prospect of her having another child (in the past she had had at least two – one died and the other(s) taken into care) as she was 55 and past her menopause. When I put it to her that she knew what she wanted was not going to happen, she dismissed this by saying 'I know *you* don't think it's going to happen, but I've seen it on the telly' (EY) and went on to relate having seen a television documentary about a 62-year-old woman having a 'test-tube' baby.

Who wants sex the most

The women were asked who wanted sex the most, them or their partners. Fourteen said that the men wanted sex more than they did, with three being very definite about this. One woman, in elaborating on her answer that it was men who wanted sex more than her, went on to explain the pressure this could lead to:

> G. [male friend, not boyfriend] kept pushing me, asking and asking. He didn't give me a break...Men think 'cos you've had a child, they think 'she's *all right*, she's easy' but they don't realise how I feel about it, I don't think they understand, you know, the feelings, the unhappiness, when you're trying to overcome it and they're just bringing it forward into your mind all the time...they just don't understand. (KN)

When I interjected (wrongly as it turned out) that the men might not know what bad experiences she had had in the past, she replied 'G. *does* know and I think he thinks I'm easy meat, but I'm not. He thinks "I'll probably get her sooner or later" but he won't' (KN).

Another of these fourteen women explained that she thought her boyfriend did want sex more than she did and that this was the case for men and women generally. But she thought that women, including her, did want sex too but that women kept the sexual feelings and desires under control:

> MM: Why do women control their sexual urges more than men?
>
> DO: Because men're silly, basically…I think women have a sort of instinct to say…they know *how* to control it and men don't really know how to control it … in a way.
>
> MM: Do you think they can't control it or they don't control it?
>
> DO: I don't think they even bother.

Two women said that they thought both they and their partners wanted sex equally. One of these women seemed to be saying that she wanted it as much as her boyfriend did but not for its own sake, rather because of the consequences for her if she did not do it: 'I think both of us. I have to go out to play with D., all the time, because of how he can be with me otherwise, which I don't like him being' (TC). Only one woman said that she thought she wanted sex more than her boyfriend but did not elaborate.

Who enjoys sex the most

One woman said that she thought she enjoyed sex more than her boyfriend but did not elaborate. Two women thought the level of enjoyment was equally shared. The remaining fourteen believed that the men they had sex with enjoyed the experience more than they did. None of the women appeared to view this as problematic or something to be challenged. Rather, it was accepted as the way things are and, indeed, this is not an uncommon view for many people in general population (Burchill 1997; Holland *et al.* 1998). Although the questions in this part of the interview were specifically asking the women about their own experiences, later they were asked about their perceptions of other people's experiences (see p.179).

Sexual abuse

Although at various points in the interviews most women had spoken of many sexual encounters in which they had not given their free and full consent, they were asked at this point specifically about sexual abuse. The reason for asking specifically about this was that although I, and others, might have labelled certain things as abusive, this was not necessarily how the women themselves always saw it. I wanted to find out what kinds of things they *did* construct as abusive and so they were asked if there had been any occasions when they had been made to do something sexual when they had not wanted to.

Only three women said that this had not happened. One of these answered the question very abruptly, immediately looked uncomfortable, asked to go to the toilet and changed the subject on her return. I interpreted this as a sign that she was uncomfortable with the topic rather than confirmation that she had never been abused. I knew that her ex-husband had used physical violence against her and that her current boyfriend was a convicted rapist. Whilst neither of these things, by definition, mean that she would have been sexually abused by them, neither are they comforting factors. For another of the three women who said they had not been abused, staff held strong suspicions that she had been sexually abused by her father when she was younger. Whether these suspicions were based on circumstantial evidence or whether she had indicated this to staff in the past, I do not know. However, she did not give any such indication to me. The third woman who said that she had not been sexually abused had certainly experienced physical violence from her boyfriend. Although their relationship was over by the time she spoke to me, because he was a fellow service user, she was finding it hard to avoid contact with him:

> KS: I just don't want him to say anything to me, I just want him to keep away, I just want him to stay out of my life, but he just won't have it at all…not at all. My mum's not very happy with him bruising me like that – my mum said 'he's not using you as a punch-bag'. My mum said he'll be for the high jump if he does it again. My brother's girlfriend said she'll come and sort him out if he don't stay away from me.

> MM: It might be better to leave it to the staff to try and sort out, because things can get a bit out of hand once families get involved.

> KS: Yeah and I end up being in the middle of it all.

Fourteen of the seventeen women had, within their own understanding of the term, been sexually abused. Five of these related one incident of abuse, although for at least two of them circumstances were such that it clearly could have happened more than once. The other nine women definitely all had multiple abusive experiences – these include several instances of abuse or prolonged abuse over time by the same man *and* different men abusing them at different times in their lives. As I note in my chapter on methodology, concepts of time, particularly of frequency and duration, can be difficult for many people with learning disabilities and researchers have to be satisfied with approximations. For the purposes of this research, exploring the types of abuse and how the women responded to it was more important to me than working out exactly how many times and when something happened.

Rather than attempt to summarise and categorise the women's experiences, as I have done so far, I think it does more justice to their histories to give a summary of each of the women and let them, as far as possible, speak in their own voices.

MC'S EXPERIENCES

MC spoke of abuse by the same man as reported in more detail by MH below, in much the same circumstances. She also reported having been raped as a child:

> MC: When I was about six or seven I was at boarding school in the country and there was a coloured lad there, he was quite tall. He pulled me into the woods and forced me down on the ground and put his penis up into me.
>
> MM: That's terrible. Did you tell anyone?
>
> MC: They said they didn't believe me.
>
> MM: Did you tell your mum and dad?
>
> MC: They said to stay away from him, but you could never avoid him.

Not being believed was a concern for this woman and was something that was raised at another point in the interview. Here I was trying to help her think through some of the potentially positive things that could happen if she reported abuse:

> MM: Well if you report the man he might get into trouble. You might get help and support. Do you think the staff would believe you?
>
> MC: No.
>
> MM: Would any of the other women on the ward believe you?
>
> MC: No.
>
> MM: Your family?
>
> MC: No.

MM: Why would nobody believe you?

MC: They just wouldn't.

MM: Do you think I would believe you?

MC: You would, yes.

MM: Well it's important to know that at least one person would believe you.

She was quite right that nobody (apart from me) believed her when she reported abuse. This was graphically illustrated by an incident that occurred during the time I was interviewing her. She had been involved in an incident with a man with learning disabilities who was kept under strict supervision at all times because of his violent behaviour but who, as part of his rehabilitation, had been allowed five minutes unsupervised time in the hospital grounds. During these few minutes MC happened to be passing and, although the details are not clear, some sexual contact took place and the man bit her face, causing extensive bruising. As she had injured herself at times of stress in the past, the staff on MC's ward maintained that this was also a self-inflicted injury, thereby obviously denying it was a bite-mark. The staff on the man's ward, however, acknowledged it was a bite and that he had inflicted it but that she had consented to the sexual contact. I made a formal complaint about the incident to the hospital management but it ended unsatisfactorily with the view (put forward by the man's (male) psychiatrist) being accepted that the man had got carried away by sexual passion.

MC also recounted an instance of having been sexually abused in a toilet by a hospital porter.

BN'S EXPERIENCES

BN did not give much detail about her experiences of abuse. In fact, she was clearly uncomfortable with talking about it and attempted to change the subject. But she did say that one of the men whom she had been in a brief relationship with (who did not have learning disabilities) and in whose flat she had stayed had made her have sex when she did not want to and when he wanted her out of the flat had pushed her down the stairs (this had been witnessed by a male friend who had mild learning disabilities). She did not say anyone else had abused her although her social worker had strong suspicions (based on her knowledge of the family) that BN's father may have sexually abused her.

EY'S EXPERIENCES

EY spoke of many different instances of having been forced to do sexual things she did not want throughout her life, beginning with sexual abuse by her father when she was a girl:

> EY: My dad had my body when I was twelve…I learned from him about sex, he used to teach me about sex and that's another reason why I'm like I am sometimes.
>
> MM: What do you mean?
>
> EY: My father said he was going to change me into a person who would go with all the men…
>
> MM: And you think that's worked in some way?
>
> EY: Yes, he said he was going to make me into a prostitute.
>
> MM: That's a terrible thing to say.
>
> EY: That's another reason why I go with the men see? Because my father changed me and I'm not so nice as I used to be, because my father done it to me. And he's not alive now, good job, but he did say he'd do something to me that would make me go with all the men.
>
> MM: Did you ever tell anybody about what your dad did?
>
> EY: I told my mum and she had him put away.

FM'S EXPERIENCES

FM was one of the women who reported a single instance of rape, in her case it was by a fellow pupil at residential college:

> FM: When I was at college, it happened there. A boy there wanted to do it and I said 'Right, A., can you stop please' and he carried on.
>
> MM: What did you do?
>
> FM: He took me by the arm behind the chairs, he asked me to lay down. I laid and the next minute, he wanted to make love with me. He decided to have sex, he grabbed two of my hands and he was pushing down very hard, very hard on the palm of my hands – he wouldn't let go. I said 'A., stop please', but I couldn't put my hand down, I said 'A., that's enough please'. It was hard for me, I couldn't move.
>
> MM: That must have been very frightening. Did you tell anybody about it afterwards?

FM: After he finished, I said 'I'm going to tell somebody of you' and I went to the office and told Mr J. The next day he took A. into the office and he got told off, because he wouldn't let go of me.

MM: That sounds very upsetting.

FM: Yes it was.

GJ'S EXPERIENCES

GJ did not give many details but said that the man with learning disabilities she regularly had sex with had made her do things she did not want to do. Another woman with more severe learning disabilities had also, in the course of my work, made similar complaints about this particular man.

TY'S EXPERIENCES

TY was another woman who said she had been forced by a man with learning disabilities to have sex at a social services hostel. She did not give many details. The man she named was known to my team as having sexually abused a number of vulnerable people. In addition, although she did not name it as abuse or exploitation herself, staff members were worried about a relationship this woman had with a man without learning disabilities. He had befriended her at a time when she was lonely and grieving over the death of her boyfriend. The man who was supposedly 'helping her get over it' initiated sexual contact with her at that time.

GN'S EXPERIENCES

GN reported a particular incident in the context of other things which had happened:

> MM: Has any man ever forced you to have sex when you didn't want to, tried to make you do it?
>
> GN: Sometimes.
>
> MM: Can you tell me what happened?
>
> GN: They force me to.
>
> MM: Who's 'they'? Residents or men from outside?
>
> GN: Residents – if you don't have sex with them, they get in a bad mood and tell you to fuck off.

MM: Yes, but that's not the same as making you do it – has anybody ever forced you to do what they want?

GN: Yes.

MM: Has that happened a lot or just once?

GN: A couple of times.

MM: Was it the same man or different men?

GN: Different men.

MM: Who were they?

GN: [no reply]

MM: It's OK if you don't want to tell me.

GN: I do! K. [hospital resident] do it, M's boyfriend, K. done it to me on the ward one day, he's rude, he pulled my knickers down in the quiet room and he put his penis into my backside and I didn't like it.

MM: Did you tell anybody about what K. did?

GN: I told the night nurse and she put him out the ward and banned him for it, stopped him coming up to the ward for a couple of nights.

MM: What did you think about that?

GN: D. [her boyfriend] heard about it and he was very cross about it.

MM: What do you think should have happened to K?

GN: I would have liked him to be told off.

MM: Who do you think should have told him off?

GN: Anybody. He did do it to me in the ward, a long time ago, I'm not lying, he pulled my nightie up, he did.

MM: I believe you.

GN: I'm not lying. He asked me did I want sex and I said no to him and he kept carrying on.

The man with learning disabilities GN is referring to was the boyfriend of MH (see below).

TC'S EXPERIENCES

Referring to her boyfriend of many years standing, the man she one day hoped to marry, TC said the following (she calls sex 'playing with'):

A man has forced me to play with him, because of what he is with me otherwise, D. did that. I've had to go out to him, to satisfy him that's all, to keep him happy, to stop him from going for me. That's what I have to do.

MH'S EXPERIENCES

MH described only one incident with a man with learning disabilities in hospital but she was thought by staff to have been abused by her boyfriend (a different man with learning disabilities) on numerous occasions. Although she does not relate any of that here when asked the specific question about abuse (perhaps suggesting it is harder to recognise abuse and name it when it happens by a loved one), at other times during my work with her she complained at length about her boyfriend's sexual behaviour. But here she is talking about a different man:

> MM: Did you want to have sex with S.?
>
> MH: No, I wasn't pleased with it, he locked me in the shed, I didn't want to do it in the shed, it's dirty in the shed. He said 'do it in the shed, like it or lump it'. I tried to get out of the door and I couldn't, the door was locked. He said 'if you kick that door down, you'll pay for it'.
>
> MM: That all sounds very upsetting. Do you know if he did that to anyone else?
>
> MH: He used to hurt all the women.
>
> MM: Yes, lots of women have complained to me about him.

The man she is referring to was well known to me (not personally, as I had never met him, but by reputation) as many women had complained to me about him. He did have a key to the shed, which he had had access to as part of his job in the hospital. I made official complaints about him to the (male) psychiatrist responsible for his care but was treated disrespectfully by him and my concerns described as exaggerated. Illustrating that not all staff in learning disability services take issues of sexual abuse seriously (McCarthy and Thompson 1996), this psychiatrist told me that lots of men in the hospital behaved as S. did so it would be unfair to pick on him and this would make him angry. When I took my complaints (the original one about S. and new ones about the doctor) to the hospital managers, there was an investigation of sorts but it was not resolved to my satisfaction. At the time of writing (some

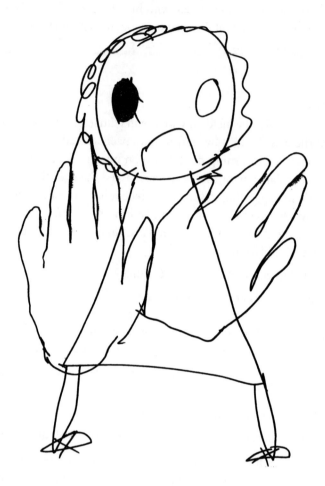

Figure 4.5

three or four years later), reports about S.'s abusive sexual behaviour towards women with learning disabilities are still emerging.

HC'S EXPERIENCES

HC was one of the least able and least communicative of the woman in the study and did not give much detail about what had happened to her:

MM: Has anyone ever forced you to have sex when you didn't want to?

HC: J. [hospital resident] did once, he done it to me once, he just wanted to do it.

MM: Did you tell anybody about that?

HC: No I didn't tell anybody, no.

MM: Do you know why you didn't tell anybody?

HC: I didn't tell the staff, no.

MM: What do you think the staff would have done?

HC: They might have had a word with him.

LT'S EXPERIENCES

LT related her experience of sexual abuse by a neighbour when she was young and unwelcome attempts by boys at school:

> LT: Yes, where I used to live, the man four doors down, Mr T. I was 14 and he called me into his garage and told me to take my trousers down. So I said no, but he did it, he put his finger, the index finger...how can I put this...? He put his finger inside me. I was frightened to death, I didn't know what to do.
>
> MM: That's really horrible, so what happened?
>
> LT: I told police and he got arrested.
>
> MM: That was very brave of you to tell.
>
> LT: It's put me off sex for life...When I was younger at school, boys used to try to force me in the bushes to do it, but I wouldn't let them do it. I was too young.

DO'S EXPERIENCES

DO had had two abusive episodes in her life (at the time of interviewing she was still only nineteen years old, the youngest woman in the study):

> MM: Has anyone ever forced you to have sex when you didn't want to?
>
> DO: Yes, my dad when I was younger, about 13 I think, he was doing things that didn't make me...I knew it was wrong, but he forced me into doing it.
>
> MM: Did you tell anybody about it?
>
> DO: It wasn't easy...My dad told me not to tell anybody, because if I did tell anyone, he'd beat me, so I had no choice really. It was only when me

and my dad were left on our own he did it, when anyone else was there, it was all family love and all that. I really wanted to tell my mum but I couldn't. I knew if I told my mum she wouldn't believe me anyway and it would all go through police and everything and I didn't want that.

MM: Last week you mentioned that you had been raped...were you referring to what happened with your dad?

DO: No, that was an old bloke I knew. Me and other kids used to help him with the paper round, he used to give us £1 each. All the kids used to do it, but they stopped and I carried on and he started on me, getting all these funny ideas. It was *all right* for a little while, then he got a job at a playschool, clearing up and he asked me would I help and I thought 'Why not?'. It would give me a bit of extra money and that's when it all started with him, down there. That's why my mum and dad stopped me from going out, they wouldn't let me out of the house, not even for five minutes.

MM: So you told your mum and dad about it?

DO: Yes and my dad went absolutely loopy, he started getting all his mates with all these baseball bats...

MM: Did anybody tell the police?

DO: No, we had enough trouble as it was with the police, I'm scared of them because they came around and arrested my dad before.

MM: How old were you when this happened with the old man?

DO: Sixteen. He cornered me into a corner and I didn't have my chance to get away. He didn't listen and that made it harder on me. And now there's another bloke, around here, one of the blokes that knew my dad, said to me to go with him in his car and go for a dirty weekend. I said 'No way, I'm not going out with you, you're too old, you're old enough to be my father'.

MM: You've obviously had some bad experiences with men. Has it affected your attitude to men generally?

DO: It makes me anxious when I'm walking down the street and there's a man behind me...'cos you don't know what they're like...Some men are nice and some are really, really horrible.

MM: When you had your bad experiences, did you have anyone to help you get over them?

DO: No, I had to do it all myself. But my friend E. has had the same experiences and I have spoken to her about it...we hang around together.

MM: Do you have any thoughts about why men do those things to girls?

DO: Because they're stupid basically, aren't they? I don't know why they do it, they must be bored I suppose.

MM: Well, I don't know about that...if you're bored you could read a book or watch telly, you don't have to go and rape somebody.

DO: I don't know why they do it, there's no need for it is there? Is it fun or what? I mean what's the attraction of hurting other people?

TD'S EXPERIENCES

TD did not give much detail but related an instance of having been taken to the shed in the hospital and having to do something she did not like. She had also, in another hospital, been touched in a sexual way by a man with learning disabilities whilst walking in the grounds. She had complained to staff about this incident and that had prompted the referral to me.

KN'S EXPERIENCES

KN had also had two episodes of abuse in her life. First, she talks about how she was raped by her father as a girl, eventually having his child when she was seventeen and how her brothers were initially suspected of abusing her:

KN: My brothers sent the police to the hospital when I had P. and said to my dad 'we have been accused of K. being pregnant, but dad it's you'. My dad told me if I didn't keep my mouth shut, he'd be in prison. I didn't understand. When my mum came to see me I told her what they said and she said 'it's right, he'll go to prison and I will have to go in prison as well'. I said 'why you, you ain't done nothing wrong?' and she said 'I will have to go in prison because I wasn't watching you, it's called "aiding and abetting"'. I didn't grasp it, but I didn't say nothing. I think my mum felt guilty until the day she died, because she apologised to me. I said to her 'you haven't got nothing to be sorry for'.

MM: How did your brothers know it was your dad?

KN: Because they didn't make me pregnant and he kept blaming them.

MM: But how did they know it was him and not anybody else?

> KN: Because P. looks dead like him. I think that with my dad is what's put me off sex and I try not to let him see that I'm hurting. He's so much like my dad, but it's not his fault. It's really sad. I feel guilty all the time, but I know it's not my fault.

As well as this earlier traumatic experience, she later had another abusive experience with a man who also had mild learning disabilities:

> I had another boyfriend, he took me in the woods, he said there's some pretty animals there and me, being young in the mind, thought 'that's good, I like animals'. But I never dreamt he was going to rape me, I didn't realise it was called rape, I ran away, I don't know how I got home and told my Mum and Dad what happened. He worked with my stepdad and my uncle. They got him on the side and said 'You mustn't do that. We know you're not sensible, but you're not to do that, you've scared her now'. My mum told me to tell him to look for another girlfriend and I did. I didn't go out with him any more. That was 10 or 20 years ago now. (KN)

In addition to their own experiences, which are extensive, seven women knew of others who had also been sexually abused. Six of these women knew other women with learning disabilities that this had happened to – all apart from one were other women in hospitals. This suggests that the institutional 'grapevine' carries these stories between women with learning disabilities in hospitals in a way that does not happen so readily in community services where people with learning disabilities are more isolated from one another. In terms of confidentiality for the individuals concerned this may be bad, but in terms of forging some sense of solidarity or shared experience between women there is a positive side to it.

One woman knew that her boyfriend (without learning disabilities) had been sexually assaulted by another man. One woman who said that she had not been abused herself did not know of anyone else who had been but said that her boyfriend may well abuse other people: 'P. doesn't know what he's doing half the time, he's out of control, he'll have it with anybody' (TM). This man had, in fact, been referred to my team for sexually abusing less able women.

As well as giving information about what happened to them and how they felt about it, some of the women also revealed – in passing, mostly – what happened to the men who abused them. Aside from the woman who said that her father was imprisoned for what he did to her and the woman whose neighbour was arrested (but very likely not prosecuted), it is apparent that there were no legal consequences for all the other men. Two of the fathers who raped their daughters were not reported to the police because of the perceived trouble that would cause in the wider family network; another man who raped was not reported because the woman's family were known to the police and wanted no further dealings with them. The most likely response to men with learning disabilities was, if anything at all happened, to be 'told off'. The man with learning disabilities who attacked MC and bit her face was already on sexual suppressant medication because of his past abusive behaviour. The doctor's response to his latest offence was to increase the dose of this medication and keep him on the ward for two days. See Chapter Six for a fuller discussion on achieving justice for women who have been sexually abused.

Whether the women themselves had sexually abused others

It seemed unlikely, from what the women had said about not taking the initiative and often not wanting or enjoying sexual contact, that they would have sexually abused anyone else, but, nevertheless, they were asked about this. Somewhat surprisingly, only one woman appeared offended by the question and so answered in a rather indignant tone of voice. The others all gave matter-of-fact, short answers to the effect that they did not do this. Occasionally, there was a brief elaboration:

I've never forced anybody, they only force me. (EY)

No, I'm not the forcing type. (MH)

One woman initially said that she had, in fact, forced a man to have sex with her, so this was explored further. It transpired that her definition of her forcing him was: 'I kept on at him until he said yes' (GN). Although this was, as I pointed out to her, a form of pressure and, therefore, unacceptable, it was not the same as forcing someone. At an earlier stage in the interview this woman had said that she did not ask men for sex. Therefore, there was some inconsistency in what she said regarding this.

Sex with less able people

Because it would be naïve to expect people to freely admit to sexually abusing others, I tried another way of gauging whether the women would do this or take advantage of others sexually by asking them about sex with people less able than themselves. It is worth noting here that although I meant a lesser intellectual ability, the women themselves, as often as not, constructed 'less able' in physical terms – that is, people in wheelchairs were mentioned a number of times, as were people who could not talk. Through further clarification from me, such as 'people who are not as clever as you' or 'people who can't understand things like you do', and by naming certain individuals known to both of us as examples, I was satisfied that the women had grasped I was talking about intellectual and not just physical disabilities (although for some of the people we had in mind, both may have been present). In this part of the interview I had to use language I would normally avoid because of its stigmatising nature – for example, 'handicapped people' – as these were terms the women themselves used freely and understood.

With reference to the question of whether they had, or would have, sex with someone less able than themselves, two women did not respond and one response was very unclear. Of the remaining fourteen, two women said that they might have sex with less able men if the men asked them to. One of these mentioned a specific man who used a wheelchair and who was intellectually quite able and who I knew did initiate sexual contact with others. However, by far the biggest majority (twelve) said that they would not do this. Moreover, they felt this was a wrong thing to do because it was 'not fair':

> No, it's not fair on the handicapped ones, because they wouldn't know what's going on. (LT)

> I think it's terrible, I really do, especially if they're not right upstairs [points to head]. (KN)

> No, oh no, poor buggers, it'd kill them, wouldn't it? (EY)

It is interesting that a number of the women saw it as being unfair and saw less able people, by definition, as being at a disadvantage. This is similar to the view taken by many professionals and academics (Brown and Turk 1992; McCarthy and Thompson 1998). What is interesting is that the women themselves very frequently had sex with men more able than themselves – in effect, they were the less able people in those encounters. But they did not usually describe their own experiences as being unfair on those grounds.

In the course of the above discussions three of the women (all in hospitals, reinforcing my earlier point regarding an institutional 'grapevine') said that they knew of men who did have sex with less able people and that they thought this was wrong:

> What makes them want to have sex with a person with a discapability [sic]? I think it's all bloody wrong. (MC)

EY: Some of the men do, some of the patients and some of the outside men.

MM: They chose the handicapped ones?

EY: If they can't get a high-grade patient, they get a low-grade.

MM: What do you think about that? Is it all right?

EY: No. I've talked to people about that, I don't think it is right.

MM: I agree, but why do you think it's bad to have sex with a handicapped person?

EY: Because it could kill them or send them silly.

MM: Do you think they understand enough about sex?

EY: No they don't and it's not their fault, it's the person who goes with them.

MM: I think you're right and if you ever know this is happening you should report it, because those people need others to look out for them.

Sex education

The women were asked how they first learned about sex. As is apparent at various points in this study, the women had clearly been influenced by many of the various 'messages' that are in circulation about sexual matters, many of which are sexist and damaging (Millard 1994). I was, therefore, interested in some of the subtle ways sexual messages are communicated but this did not prove to be a fruitful area to explore, probably because of the abstract nature of the subject matter. Consequently, the emphasis here is on formal and informal sex education and learning from experience.

Three women did not answer this question, although one said that she had not learned anything about sex at school. Three women said that they first learned by being sexually abused as children or young women – two by their fathers and one by an older pupil at school. One of these went on to receive some formal sex education many years later but the other two did not. Women with learning disabilities learning about sex through being abused is noted elsewhere in the literature (Hard and Plumb 1987). Five other women also learned from direct experience, some of which was consented sex – for example, 'I went out with a bloke called T., quite a few years ago and he taught me' (BN). For two of these five women, their consent is in doubt:

MM: How did you first learn about sex?

TY: When T. did it to me.

No one told me, except my boyfriend wanted it. I still have to go to him.
(TC)

Only five of the women said that they had received any formal or structured
sex education. Three had had some education at school (all special schools
for children with mild/moderate learning disabilities) and two had been
taught at adult education (one adult education programme in hospital and
one at an Adult Training Centre). Two did not say what the content was,
whilst three of these women specified that they had only been taught about
reproduction and contraception (this is still a common feature of sex education offered to non-disabled young people at school (Holland *et al.* 1998):

DO: We used to break up in groups – girls in one class and boys in
another. They told us what sort of things to use, contraception and that,
what to do if you are pregnant, things like that.

MM: So, it sounds like it's mostly about pregnancy – did they talk about
feelings, good sex, bad sex.

DO: Not really, they didn't go that deep.

One woman who had been taught about reproduction made a point of saying that she had not understood what she had been taught, despite the fact
that she had what might be considered an advantage over the other students
because she had already given birth to a child herself. The importance of sustaining sex education input over time and/or returning to it periodically to
remind and reinforce earlier messages is illustrated by this woman. Despite
having had a child and previous sex education, she gave the impression that
she was learning some basic messages from me for the first time:

You've given me a lot of things to think about…when you showed me
those pictures, when you said you don't have to conceive and have a
child…if you do it this way, but not that way…I didn't realise any of that
until you showed me…so I learnt something there. (KN)

The most common source of information about sex (for eight women) was
when it came informally from other women. Six women named their mothers
(including one foster mother), one a younger sister and one woman friend as
having talked to them about sex. In seven of the eight cases the subject matter
was, as one woman put it, 'the facts of life' (TM) – that is, purely concerned
with menstruation, pregnancy and contraception:

MM: What did your mum tell you?

TM: Monthly periods, nine-month labour, all the pain, caesareans.

Only one woman had been spoken to about other, less biological, matters – this was a young woman who had been placed with foster parents because of sexual and physical abuse at home and her foster mother had talked with her about her experience of rape.

Despite mothers being a more forthcoming source of information than anyone else, two women pointed out that their mothers had not talked to them about sex at all. One said that her mother had not told her anything specifically 'because of what I suffer with' (TC), although she was referring to her epilepsy rather than her learning disability. For the other woman it was because her mother was uncomfortable with any discussion of sexual matters and, she seems to imply, was uneducated herself:

> When I told my mum about the sex education, she said 'I'm as green as grass, I should come with you'. But my mum didn't like talking about it… if she saw a newspaper with a woman showing her…she didn't like it, she'd turn the page quick. If there was anything in the paper about abused women or anything like that, she'd say not to read it. (KN)

Other people's sexual experiences

The women were asked what they knew, or thought, about other people's sexual experiences. I was interested in how they perceived the sexuality of non-disabled people so asked them specifically about this, suggesting, by way of examples, that they thought about people who did not live or work in the same places as them – for example, their families, staff and their families, etc. The women were asked three related questions: whether they thought other people did have sex; whether they thought this was broadly the same as theirs or not; and whether they generally thought men and women enjoyed sex equally.

Two women did not know whether other people had sex and one thought they did not. The remaining fourteen thought other people did have sex, although a number of them pointed out that it was difficult to know and/or that they were not sure:

> That's quite a hard question actually. (FM)

> I don't know, do I? I'm not there. (GJ)

These women were highlighting the difficult nature of the questions, which essentially required them to use their imagination and/or extrapolate from their own experiences, things which are often hard for people with learning disabilities. Not surprisingly, then, six women did not know or could not imagine whether other people would have broadly the same kind of sexual experiences as they did. However, eleven women did venture an opinion, with two of them thinking other people's sex would be like their own and nine thinking it would be different. Seven of the nine gave reasons why they thought it would be different, including use of different sexual positions, having privacy, having sex at night instead of during the day. One woman, who had experienced sex inside and outside of hospital, thought her own sex life outside hospital was closer to the 'norm' than what she was currently experiencing in hospital. Frequency of sexual contact seemed to be the essential difference: 'Sex life is different here. At home it was more now and again, not all the time like it is here' (TM).

As to their thoughts on how other people enjoyed their sexual activity, one woman did not know and four thought women and men would both enjoy sex equally. Three women, however, thought that women generally enjoyed sex more than men. Two of them believed this was because love and marriage meant women would enjoy sex more. Nine women thought that it was men who enjoyed sex the most, although one added the rider that sometimes women could enjoy it too and gave the example of her married niece, who, she thought, liked sex. None of the women knew why they thought it was men who enjoyed sex the most: 'they just would really' (DO) was the general feeling. It is reasonable to assume that many of them were basing this on their own experience. Indeed, one woman said as much:

MM: Why would men enjoy it more than women?

TC: I know why – because of my boyfriend enjoying.

The women's belief in, and acceptance of, the fact that men simply did enjoy sex more than women concerned me and led to the following conversation with one of the most able women:

MM: Thinking generally about other people, who enjoys sex the most?

DY: Men.

MM: Why is that?

DY: Don't really know, do I? Men *do* enjoy it more than women.

MM: That's what most people say, but I think it's important to think why that is.

DY: [irritated, exasperated tone] How do *I* know why?

MM: I'm not saying you do know, or that *I* know either, but it's important to think about, because I don't think it's good enough. I think both women and men should enjoy it equally and it bothers me that they don't.

DY: [flippant tone of voice] Does it?

MM: Yes. Do you think it's important? Does it bother you that men get more pleasure than women?

DY: It don't really bother me anyway [big obvious yawn].

Her apparent lack of concern about the situation irritated me, just as my concern irritated her and, as the atmosphere was becoming tense, I dropped the subject.

Sex on television

One woman did not watch TV and another gave an answer totally unconnected to the question and seemed not to want to discuss it. The remaining fifteen had all seen some sexual activity on TV. Only two reported any embarrassment watching it. I asked whether what they saw bore any relation to what they had experienced themselves. Despite the fact that they only had to remember what they had seen (as opposed to the previous questions which asked them to think hypothetically), this seemed a very difficult question. Ten women said that they did not know or did not answer. Of the five who did know, all of them thought the sex they saw on TV was very different from their own. Three did not say how and two did – one said sex on TV was much more passionate than real life; the other said people on TV had sex lying down and they kissed and cuddled, none of which she did.

The women were asked whether men and women on TV enjoyed sex equally and all fifteen answered this question – two thought both enjoyed it equally; six thought men enjoyed it more; and six thought women enjoyed it more. Of those who thought men got most pleasure, only one woman could say why and she went on to describe a rape scene. Of those who thought women got more pleasure, all gave reasons and these varied considerably: one said she knew the women liked it because they verbally encouraged the men and made noises; two thought the women on TV liked it because they were married and wanted babies (whether this was actually part of the plot of programmes they were thinking of or their own projection I do not know); one thought the women on TV enjoyed it because if they did not, the men would force them anyway; and one thought she could tell the women on TV enjoyed sex more than the men because they stayed in bed, looking relaxed, while the men got dressed and went home. The fifteenth woman gave one of those answers which made me realise that, as researchers, we sometimes ask stupid questions. She pointed out that neither the women nor the men on TV enjoyed having sex because they were not really doing it, they were only acting!

Although I did not specifically ask about it, three women said that they knew that their boyfriends watched pornographic videos or had magazines. Two women did not mind and one of these thought it might be a useful educational tool: 'It won't do them any harm, it might show them different ways with *their* women' (BN). The third woman did mind:

DY: D's [boyfriend] got them upstairs in his bedroom.

MM: Do you watch them?

DY: No, but I did see them when I was younger.

MM: What did you think of them?

DY: Disgusting.

MM: Do you mind your boyfriend watching them?

DY: I do, yeah, I don't like him watching them, other women having sex with men and that...

MM: Have you told him that you don't like him seeing them?

DY: Yeah.

MM: What did he say?

DY: Not much really.

MM: Does he still watch them?

DY: Yeah.

What the women liked about their bodies

Several related questions were asked to try to find out how the women felt about themselves as adult women, their body image and appearance. They were first asked what they liked about their own bodies. Despite this being a

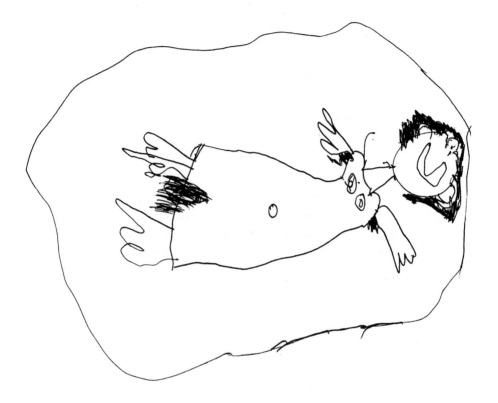

Figure 4.6 'I like my body'

simple question in linguistic terms, it proved difficult to answer for several of the women and a number asked for clarification.

Four women said that there was nothing they liked about their bodies and a further three said that it was 'all right' but could not or did not say anything positive beyond that. Most of the remaining nine women needed a fair amount of prompting to say what they liked. This was unusual, compared with the rest of the interviews as a whole, so it may mean that what they said reflected their wish to give me an answer rather than being a true reflection of how they really felt about their bodies.

Nevertheless, three women were mostly positive, listing a number of features they liked about themselves:

MM: I want to ask now how you feel about your body. Not sexual parts necessarily, but your body generally. What do you like about your body?

EY: I like my figure [laughs].

MM: Good. What is it you like about your figure?

EY: It's nice and soft, you know, but I am a bit fat, but it's a nice built body, nice backside and different things.

MM: OK, anything else you like?

EY: My feet and my legs. That lady in the chiropodist told me I had nice feet. I don't want to be rude or nothing, but when I was going with my boyfriend he told me I had nice legs.

Another of these women said that she liked her legs, despite the fact that she had very bad leg ulcers which she had aggravated for months by picking at them. The medical staff were of the opinion that she did not want the ulcers to get better and so was making sure they did not. One perceived explanation for this, put forward by the medical and nursing staff, was that this behaviour was linked to her emotional and mental health problems.

Six women could, after some prompting, come up with one or two things about their bodies which they liked. The list is interesting for its content and variety – one woman said she liked her face and two others their figures. But after that the list becomes a bit more unusual – one woman said that she liked her nose (she made exaggerated claims about how small and delicate hers was and how big and ugly mine was!); another woman said what she liked about her body was how clean it was (in fact, she had grave problems with her personal hygiene); another said that what she liked was her body 'being left alone' (TC). What these responses demonstrate is that it is not really possible to talk about women's bodies in straightforward and positive terms without tapping into more complicated issues.

What the women disliked about their bodies

Not surprisingly, in view of the above, the women found these questions easier to answer and less clarification and prompting were necessary. However, four women still did not know or reply. Two women were negative about almost everything about the way they looked, although one of these was overwhelmingly concerned about her weight. She felt that being fat overshadowed any other, positive features she might have: 'I think "look at you, you've got a nice face, but your body's fat and horrible"' (KN). As with so many women (Orbach 1978; Szekely 1988), her perception did not match reality – I think she could have been described, at most, as slightly over-weight. Six women listed one or two negative features about their bodies – two of these also concerned perceived excess weight and one said that she thought she was too tall. Two women said that they disliked their genital area – one specified that she disliked the way her pubic hair got itchy when she had sex and the other linked her dislike of her genitals to her dislike of sex.

One woman, who was prone to exaggeration, nevertheless obviously did not like the shape of her body (she had Prader-Willi Syndrome and was short and overweight):

> I don't like the smallness of my hands and feet and my arms and legs aren't long enough. My legs can't take my weight and I get tired. I don't get enough air in my lungs because I'm so short. I don't get as much oxygen as tall people. (MC)

Four women said that there was nothing about their bodies which they dis-liked (although three of these later said there were things they wanted to change – see below). One of the women who said that there was nothing she disliked had a lot of facial hair. As this is something most women do not like and about which there are strong social taboos (Brownmiller 1986), I would have liked to have discussed this further. However, I felt it had to be raised by the woman herself as it would have been tactless for me to draw attention to it. In the event she did not mention it and it was, therefore, not discussed. (See McCarthy 1998 for a fuller discussion of this.)

What the women wanted to change about their bodies

The women were asked *if* they could, what they would change about the way they looked. Two did not know. Another two wanted to change everything. One of these (whose Prader-Willi Syndrome meant she had no secondary sexual characteristics or womb) spoke very movingly about the profound changes she wished for.[3]

---

3   It should be noted that this statement came from her after I had had several sex education sessions with her, which almost definitely accounts for the fact that she mentions the clitoris: 'I'd change the way I was born, so I could be born again a normal female baby and I'd have a clitoris and breasts when I was older and I'd see my periods and be able to have kids and not have diabetes' (MC).

Four other women wanted to change specific things, such as strengthening weak ankles or have longer hair. Two of these women specifically mentioned cosmetic surgery – one wanted facial surgery so she could be made 'as beautiful as some of them on the telly' (EY) and the other wanted a breast enlargement, despite having very large breasts already. This was the woman with mental health problems mentioned above regarding her leg ulcers. I did have the feeling that she said that she wanted even larger breasts to get some kind of reaction from me, but this may be pure projection on my part as I find it hard to believe that someone with very large breasts would want them even bigger.

By far the most common desired change (named by ten of the fourteen women who said that they wanted to change something) was to lose weight. This accurately reflects the preoccupations of most non-disabled women (Lawrence 1987), suggesting that women with learning disabilities are similarly affected by social pressures to be thin. One woman who was very thin described the responses of other young women to her: 'Everybody at college says to me "I wish I had your figure". They all say "You're so lucky"' (DO). Most women did not specify how much they wanted to lose but the two who did had unrealistic and worryingly low target rates of seven or eight stone. Some of the women seemed more distressed about their size and more serious about losing weight than others, but all were concerned. Many spoke of how difficult it was to actually lose weight and how their desire to be thinner conflicted with their enjoyment of food ('I like my food' (MC)) or their need to eat ('I would not like to be fat, but I have to eat. I have to eat to live, I do' (TC)).

Three women spoke explicitly about how staff in learning disability services influenced or controlled their decisions about weight. My wider knowledge of the services would suggest this was a more common issue than it appears from these numbers, however. One woman said that it was her keyworker's decision that she should diet, not her own. Another described the staff's efforts to control her eating in the following way: 'They won't let me have ice-cream. They say "you can't have this, you can't have that". They boss me around' (MH). This woman had, in fact, put on a lot of weight as a direct result of the medication which staff had prescribed for her.

Another described how staff could exert a more subtle, but still powerful, influence as role models:

KS: I'd like to be skinny.

MM: Why do you want to be skinny?

KS: I'd like to lose a bit more.

MM: Do other people talk to you about losing weight?

KS: We're supposed to be weighed every month.

MM: Do the staff encourage you to lose weight?

KS: Yeah, I've seen the staff lose weight.

MM: The staff lose weight themselves do they?

KS: Yes, we've got these scales at the moment.

MM: Which staff lose weight?

KS: It's women staff.

MM: And do you want to be like them?

KS: Yes, 'cos we've got the scales.

As well as the influence of staff, the woman also implies that the very existence of scales in the house exerts its own form of pressure.

Whether the women's bodies gave them any pleasure

The women were asked whether their bodies were sources of pleasure for them and this was explained in two ways: either in the physical sense or psychological pleasure – for example, pride in their bodies or a more general sense of being pleased with them. Once again, this proved to be a difficult question with a number of women needing clarification. Three women did not know or give a reply. Two said that everything about their bodies felt good to them. Five women mentioned one or two specific things they got pleasure from: one said her hands because of all the things she could do with them; interestingly (although it is probably due to sexuality being the main topic of my work with the women), all the four others said that it was their sexual or private body parts which gave them some pleasure. One of these women specified that the pleasure she got was from knowing her boyfriend liked 'playing with me' (TC). The biggest single group (of six women) said that they got no good feelings at all from their bodies.

Personal hygiene

As another way of finding out how the women valued their bodies and what control they had over them, a number of questions were asked about personal hygiene. First, the women were asked whether they valued cleanliness – that is, whether it was important to them to keep clean. All said yes and this is not surprising, given how difficult it would have been for them to have said no, even if this were the case. However, it is, perhaps, worth noting that two of the women did, in fact, have very poor personal hygiene, despite being considered by their support staff as being quite capable of attending to their own needs (see below for further discussion). What was interesting was the reasons the women gave for why it was important to keep clean. Five gave expected responses such as unpleasant body odour and related social consequences and some emphasised the importance of paying particular attention to hygiene at certain times: 'I have a bath to keep clean. Because us ladies have private parts and ladies' problems [in a low voice], periods, you've got to be careful of that and have a bath' (FM).

But an equal number named dire physical consequences ranging from the general (sores, illnesses and diseases) to the specific (whooping cough, bronchitis and AIDS). Because of the exaggerated and incorrect nature of much of these responses, I think it is likely that the women may have been warned by carers that they could get some kind of infection if they did not keep clean and they had then associated this with the names of any illnesses they knew of.

The women were asked about their access to bathrooms – that is, whether they could have as many baths, showers and washes as they wanted. Rather surprisingly (given that all except one woman lived with groups of others where there were often far more people than bathrooms), all the women said that there were no restrictions on them – at most a few women said that they had to wait their turn but none suggested this was for unreasonable lengths of time. If this is an accurate reflection, learning disability services are certainly managing this aspect of people's care very well in less than ideal circumstances.

The women were asked whether they had complete control over their own personal hygiene or whether staff or their carers played a role. Five women said that others did play a role, which usually involved the woman being told when to have a bath or a wash. In four cases this was staff and for one woman it was her mother (with whom she did not live). Sometimes, this advice or instruction was accepted by the women concerned and, sometimes, it was resented, with the women asserting that they were old enough or capable enough to see to themselves. Some women distanced themselves from others in their peer group, whom they described as 'dirty' or 'too lazy' to attend to their own personal hygiene, or because they were simply not as competent as them: 'I'm more sensible than her, I can do it, she's the same age as me, but they have to wash her' (MH).

One woman said that the staff did not try to influence her personal hygiene and that she took care of herself. This was one of the very few instances when I knew a woman was not telling the truth. She had, in fact, very poor personal hygiene, especially during her periods, and staff certainly did play an active role in trying to get her to change her habits. I did discuss this with her at a later stage of my work (therefore, the conversation was not recorded or transcribed as the interviews were). She was not a verbally articulate woman and so it was hard to be sure exactly what she felt. But my interpretation of what was going on was that refusing to wash or change her clothes was, for her, a way of gaining some control over her own life and, importantly, a weapon to annoy and upset the staff. Using your body as a 'weapon' when you are otherwise powerless to exert control over your situation is well recognised in many diverse contexts, such as eating disorders (MacLeod 1981), self-harm (Burstow 1992) and political protests (Campbell et al. 1994).

Only two women mentioned shaving their legs and underarms (nobody was specifically asked about this). Both said that they could not do this for themselves and one relied on staff and one on her mother to do this for them. For both, shaving was not a choice but a perceived necessity: 'You've got to, you can't leave it, can you?' (KS).

For the other woman the messages about getting rid of body hair had been internalised to the point where she saw it as an essential part of being a woman:

> MM: Why do women shave their legs and underarms?
>
> MH: I think it's more better if you have smooth legs.
>
> MM: Well lots of women do it, most do. But why do we do it?
>
> MH: Because we're women, aren't we? Men don't do it, don't have to do it. But we're not men, are we? We're ladies, we have to shave under our arms and our legs otherwise we wouldn't be human would we?

Although most of the women did not have staff explicitly telling them when and how often to wash, there were other ways staff intruded on the women's sense of themselves or their sense of personal space. For one woman, this was when staff made personal comments about her appearance:

> MM: You said before that staff didn't like your hair?

MH: No, they didn't like it when I had blonde highlights, they said I look like a tart.

MM: Who said that?

MH: One of the staff, I don't like looking like a tart.

MM: You don't. I thought it looked nice.

For another woman, staff literally intruded upon her private space:

DY: Like this morning I was just about to get in the shower and the staff came in and told me to have a bath and they saw me stark naked without any clothes on and that it was really embarrassing for me, they just looked at me while I was stark naked and it was very embarrassing. They came in and said 'you know full well you're not allowed to have a shower, you've got to have a bath' and they saw me stark naked and it was embarrassing for me.

MM: Didn't they knock on the door?

DY: No, they just peered around the door and looked at me, while I was stark naked.

MM: Can you complain to anyone about that?

DY: I will complain if it happens again.

MM: Are there no locks on the doors?

DY: Not by the showers, in case you have an accident or something.

MM: But if the staff can just walk in, so can other residents, the male residents...[4]

DY: The system in this hospital is very poor indeed, very poor.

MM: I'd complain if I were you, because it's not right.

Clothes

The women were asked questions about how they felt about the way they dressed and who had control over this. In terms of what they put on each day, almost all the women said that they decided for themselves. Some had the advice of staff in this, most did not. However, some staff made uninvited comments: 'I decide myself, but the staff like you to change sometimes, they say "I don't like that on you, change it"' (EY, aged 55).

4   Men with histories of sexual offending are on this ward.

The picture was quite different when it came to choosing what clothes to buy. Only two women had complete control over this and made all their own decisions. For one of these this was not her choice but resulted from her mother's death a few years previously – prior to that she had relied on her mother's advice when shopping, a situation she preferred. Nine women did make choices about what to buy but did so with staff help, which most wanted and appreciated. One of these women was being actively encouraged by staff to go out and shop alone and she was proud of her recent achievements in this area. For the remaining five women, staff were also involved but the balance was different: the staff chose the clothes with the women's help, as opposed to the other way around. Interestingly, this group, who played a smaller part in choosing their own clothes, were not, on the whole, less able than the other women – indeed, three of them were amongst the most able in the whole sample. What they had in common was that they were all in hospital. However, it is not possible to draw clear conclusions from this as five of the nine women who had more control over their shopping were also hospital residents. It is probably more likely to be dependent on attitudes of individual staff members rather than anything else.

Six women, from both the groups which involved some staff help, clearly expressed that staff did, in fact, have the ultimate control in the decision-making process. I asked them what would happen if they saw something *they* liked but the staff member did not. Two said that they would allow themselves to be persuaded not to buy it and four were clear that they simply would not be allowed to have it. It should not be thought that all the women were happy with staff having so much influence. In fact, this was one of the few occasions when a significant proportion (a quarter) expressed resentment towards staff and indicated that they did not always co-operate:

> I like choosing my own clothes, my nurses never let me choose my own, they like choosing them for me. (TC)

> I choose my own. The staff do say things sometimes like 'I don't think you should wear that', but it's my own decision, if I want to wear it, I will. They can't really tell me what to put on. (DO)

> Well, it's up to me, it's my money, isn't it? If I like it and they don't like it, it's tough, isn't it? If I like it, I buy it. (DY)

None of the women said that the way they dressed made them feel generally bad about themselves. Three did not give a reply and two said that they just felt 'all right' about the way they looked. Four said that the way they felt depended, largely, on whether they thought they looked fat in certain clothes. Several women said that they kept 'best clothes' which were for parties, day trips or 'in case I go out anywhere' (TD). They recognised that they looked good and felt good in these 'best clothes' compared to their everyday wear:

> MM: You mentioned your nice red coat…what do you feel like when you wear that?
>
> MC: I feel like the Queen of Araby when I go out in that. It's a treasure to have around my shoulders.

One woman wanted to dress well to please her keyworker: 'It's very important, because J. has taken pride in me, that's the way it should be, she likes me to look nice' (FM). Another had picked up very definite ideas about what clothes were appropriate for certain occasions, as the following conversation shows:

> DY: Have you got to wear black and white to go to court?
>
> MM: No, you have to look smart, but you can wear any colour. It probably wouldn't be a good idea to wear really bright colours though, if you want to make a good impression.
>
> DY: I think it's really black and white, isn't it?
>
> MM: I don't think so.
>
> DY: You're supposed to wear black and white when you go to court, aren't you?
>
> MM: I'm not aware of that, you should wear whatever you're most comfortable in.
>
> DY: I can't always get my size though, clothes are made for people who are really slim.

Seven women said that generally they felt good about the way they dressed, although few were entirely satisfied. Several wanted more or better clothes than they had. Sometimes, their wishes were very modest: 'I need some new knickers, I might get them for my birthday' (GJ). Sometimes they were more ambitious:

> My clothes make me feel good, but they don't make me feel good enough. They don't make me feel as good as what I've seen some people in. If I had something really nice, I'd feel very good. I ain't got no fancy

clothes like some people got, like the stars on the tele, I wouldn't mind something like that. (EY)

Two of the women who said that they paid attention to their appearance and thought they looked good, dressed in ways which most people would probably consider inappropriate or sloppy – for example, summer clothes in winter, clothes that were dirty or in need of repair. In one interview I attempted to explore what I saw as this mis-match between the reality of a woman's appearance and how she saw herself. This was a mistake. The woman told me that she always wore clothes that were clean and that if anything needed mending she would get it repaired. As she was saying this, wearing a stained raincoat with several buttons missing, I questioned it. It was a very awkward moment. The look on her face and tone of voice (when she said she had lost the buttons) clearly told me that, in pointing out the real state of her clothes, I had overstepped a boundary of polite and respectful discussion. I hesitated whether to make explicit reference to what I had said and apologise for my insensitivity and decided it was better not to draw any more attention to the issue and dropped it. However, I certainly regretted my rudeness and naïvety in thinking that such an issue could be explored in the way I had imagined – that is, at my initiation rather than hers. Also, part of the awkwardness at what I had done was that I think we both realised that it was outside of my role and the context of sex education for me to have been questioning the state of her clothes. Part of the discomfort for the woman herself may also have been that the discussion also exposed a difference between me and her because my clothes were always clean and in good repair.

Sexual health

The women were asked whether they had ever had anything wrong with, or infections in, their genitals. I did not specify sexually transmitted diseases (STDs) as I anticipated (rightly as it turned out) that not all the women would have recognised when something was sexually transmitted.

I was somewhat surprised to find that the majority of women said that they had had such infections. Surprised because I simply did not know that infections of that kind were so common and because, in my sexuality work with women with learning disabilities more broadly, giving advice, information and reassurance on this particular aspect of sexual health (as opposed to HIV prevention) had not been a strong component. This is reflected in the field generally, where there is, arguably, an over-emphasis on HIV and AIDS at the expense of more common, though less serious, STDs.

Nine women said that they had had infections. Another declined to answer the question and there was a definite awkwardness or tension apparent, which led me to feel that she probably had but did not want to say. Three of the nine who did report infections had had two or three, the others only one. The infections mentioned included a very severe outbreak of herpes, genital warts, 'VD', thrush, cystitis and the less specific genital itching and pain or burning sensation on passing water. In addition, one woman had also had treatment for pre-cancerous abnormal cervical cells.

Only four of the nine women knew, or thought they knew, how they had got their infections. Two said that they got them from having sex with men who were not clean, one said that it was from her boyfriend and the fourth woman (one of the most able) said that it was from 'having too much sex' (DY). Most other women did not know how or why they had developed the infections and, across the whole sample, a number did not have any awareness of the nature of STDs. This was explained and at a later stage of my work with all the women I would have covered sexual health matters more thoroughly, although, as stated above, the emphasis was usually on HIV prevention. When I was explaining to one woman how STDs could be passed from one person to another, she asked the very pertinent question of how the very first person ever got infected then, to which I could only confess I had no idea!

It is, perhaps, worth noting that a lack of information about health and illness on a more general basis was common amongst the women. One woman was worried that she might be pregnant from an incident which had happened ten years previously; another was very concerned that she might catch a disease from her own toilet seat, even though she lived alone and nobody else used that toilet; another blamed a fellow resident for a perfectly normal process:

> TC: J. kicked me in the bottom years ago and that makes me do a number two every day, even when I don't like doing that at all.
>
> MM: Well, everyone has to go to the toilet, don't they? It's not because you were kicked.
>
> TC: Isn't it?

All these examples call for better health education for people with learning disabilities (Rodgers and Russell 1995). Some specialist materials are now emerging to meet this need (see the *Your Good Health* series from BILD 1998).

The women who had had any kind of infection in their genitals were asked how they had felt about this – in particular, whether they had been embarrassed or worried. I was interested in how the women would have coped with the social stigma still attached to STDs and other genito-urinary conditions. However, only one woman seemed to perceive this stigma and said that she had been too embarrassed to even tell her doctor. Another reported embarrassment, but this was not because of the nature of the infection (i.e. possibly related to sex) but due to having to scratch her genital area, which she knew was not socially acceptable. Two women said that they had been worried but this was because they had actually been ill and had been concerned for their health. None of the others seemed to feel particular embarrassment or stigma. In one case (where the woman had herpes) staff were concerned about her lack of embarrassment and the fact that she did not seem to feel the need to keep it a private matter.

Although they were not specifically asked, two women mentioned having had smear tests and how much they disliked this because it hurt. One of these explained how she had felt let down by a female member of staff who had accompanied her for the test: 'J. said to me "don't be a baby, it won't hurt" but it *did* hurt!' (MH). In my general work with women with learning disabilities in this area I have told the women that the test may well hurt them, but not for long, and that it is worth it because it can save them from getting really ill and hurting more later. The need to develop good policy and practice guidelines around health screening for women with learning disabilities is noted in the literature (Downs and Craft 1997; Ellison, Parker and Kitson 1998; McCarthy and Thompson 1998).

Contraception

Four women were not using any contraception – one was infertile (due to Prader-Willi Syndrome); one was presumed by staff to be infertile (as no pregnancy had ever occurred despite years of unprotected sex); one was past her menopause (but had previously had an intra-uterine device (IUD)); one had previously been on the Pill but had come off it as she was not sexually active at that time. Of the thirteen women who were using contraception, seven were on the Pill, four had the Depo-Provera injection and two had IUDs.

The fifteen who had ever used contraception were asked who had decided whether they should have it and which contraception to use. Seven said that doctors had decided, two said that their parents had decided (in fact, one of these women appeared not to even know she had an IUD), two said that staff had decided and three did not know or could not remember. Only one had made the decision for herself, a shocking fact given the relatively high levels of ability of the whole group. The one woman who had decided for herself was the youngest woman (only nineteen) yet she had the most mature and responsible attitude towards her own sexual health. Not only had she decided on her own contraception but also to use condoms for additional protection from HIV. In addition, she had actively sought and accepted what she saw as good quality advice: 'I went to the Family Planning Clinic and talked to them about it. They were really helpful, really helpful. I felt comfortable there, they make you feel part of it' (DO).

The respectful and inclusive way she was treated by the staff at the Family Planning Clinic contrasts sharply with some of the disrespectful, patronising and just downright unhelpful attitudes some of the other women in this study experienced from medics and staff in learning disability services:

> GN: They couldn't find my coil and I've got to go to hospital soon to get a new one. G. [female nurse] said to me the other night if I go with a man now and get pregnant, get a baby in my tummy, it'll be my own funeral.

> MM: That's not a very helpful thing for her to say, is it?

The thirteen current users of contraception were asked whether they were satisfied with their method and the way decisions were made about it. Six were satisfied, although one of these had numerous questions and concerns about the Depo-Provera injection and brought along a leaflet her GP had given her – it was full of very densely typed medical information, way above her reading and comprehension level. I clarified for her as best I could but told her that she probably needed more medical advice. Another woman said, when asked the direct question, that she was satisfied with her contraception but, at another point, indicated that she did not want to use contraception at all as she wanted to have a baby:

> MH: What will happen to me if I can't have children?

> MM: I'm not sure what you mean...

> MH: What would happen if I adopt one?

> MM: You wouldn't be able to adopt one.

> MH: I thought if I adopted one, I could look after it, dress it, put it in the pram and that. I'd like to have a baby. What am I going to do then?

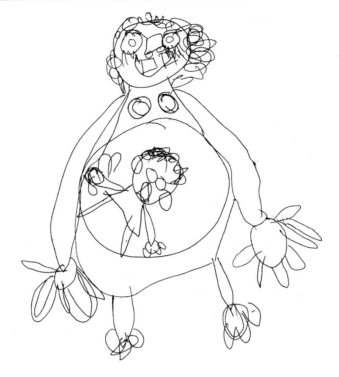

Figure 4.7

MM: Well, lots of people don't have children and I suppose you will be one of those people.

MH: I like children I do.

MM: Well, I think it's not going to happen, especially as you're already 41.

Four women were dissatisfied with their contraception. One, who had previously lived in the community but was then in hospital, complained that she was not able to make her own decision:

MM: The contraception you use now is the injection, isn't it? Whose idea was that?

TM: [long pause] We've got to here. They say it's up to you if you want it, but when the date's due and you don't want it, I mean you can't sort of say no and you've got to have it.

MM: Who makes you have it?

TM: The staff.

MM: Well if you really don't want it nobody can force you, but you're right to say that it's very hard to say no if the staff want you to...so it wasn't your choice by the sound of it and it doesn't sound like you are happy with it.

TM: I said to L.[ward manager] that I was down and depressed over not having a baby.

MM: Why do you think the staff don't want you to get pregnant?

TM: They think you can't have one here, but if I did have one on the way in nine months I would be out of here.

MM: Do you think you would be able to look after a baby?

TM: I could look after a young baby until it's beginning to walk.

MM: Then what, once it can walk?

TM: I'll still keep it, it's a strain.

MM: It is a strain. I guess a lot of staff think that you wouldn't be able to look after a baby and that's why they're concerned that you don't get pregnant.

TM: That's why they give me the injection?

MM: Yes.

The three other dissatisfied woman all wanted a different method of contraception, although only one was able to say why – she was worried about gaining weight from taking the Pill. Her mother had put her on the Pill, although the woman said that she had specifically told her that she did not want it. Two women did not know whether they were satisfied with their contraception or not.

Sense of self as sexual beings

In the final stages of the interviews I asked some questions which tried to gauge the women's sense of themselves as adult sexual beings. This was a difficult area to explore and the abstract nature of the first of these questions was clearly a struggle for some of the women. I asked each woman if she considered herself to be a sexual person – for example, someone who was interested in sex, had sexual feelings, made decisions about it, etc. – or whether sex was rather something that just happened to them. Five women did not know or reply, probably because they did not understand what I was trying to get at.

The remaining twelve, however, did reply, with the vast majority (ten) giving negative responses – that is, to the effect that they did not consider themselves to be sexual but rather that they were usually on the receiving end of someone else's sexual behaviour. This group included the woman who had been unreservedly positive about all her sexual activity and the woman who was enjoying a loving relationship with her boyfriend where she did feel in control. This indicates that there may well have been some confusion in the minds of some of the women regarding this question. However, others were crystal clear:

MC: I have no sexual feelings whatsoever.

MM: But you do have sex, so is it something you want or is it something that just happens to you?

MC: A rather lot of it is forced on me.

I don't feel as if I've got sex in my life, something holds me back, I don't know what it is, I suppose it's because of what happened to me with dad, that holds me back. And I've read about things that happen to people you know, not all women, it happens to men as well, they get strangled, get hurt, and I think to myself 'is it worth it?'. For that three minutes of madness, a lifetime of sadness. That's all it is really, isn't it? (KN)

Another woman gave an answer I found difficult to classify but feel it probably counts as a negative response as she said, when I asked her if *she* was a sexual person, 'My boyfriend likes playing with me and he should get married to me. It's not right for him to go without marrying me' (TC).

There was only one woman who gave anything approaching a positive reply, indicating that, despite negative experiences, she did consider herself to have a sexual side: 'Other people do sex to me, but I am sexy myself as well' (EY).

The women were asked a more concrete follow-up question regarding what made them feel good or bad about themselves when having sex. Four did not know and five said that they only felt bad about themselves but did not elaborate. Three women gave mixed responses: one said, for example, that during sex itself she did not feel anything much but 'at the end of it I feel brilliant. If there's any problems, we always talk about it. We kiss and make up' (DO); another woman said that how she felt about herself depended on the quality of the experience and that that, largely, depended on the man:

EY: What makes you feel good is in your body, you know, it's all lovable and that. The hard thing about it is when anybody hurts you or forces themself on you or you get any pains and that's an awful thing.

MM: Most of the time are you left feeling good about yourself or not?

EY: Sometimes good and sometimes bad, it all depends on who you go with. With some men it's always bad and with some men you think you like them and you have sex but then you don't really like them and that's a bad feeling.

MM: If you've had bad feelings with someone and he wants to have sex with you again, what would you do?

EY: It's best not to go with him.

MM: That's right, it's important to try to learn from the good and bad feelings. I think a lot of people find it difficult to learn from the bad feelings.

EY: That's true, but sometimes you have to go back again because the men say 'I'll give you a good hiding' or 'I'll make you' and they hang around and you can't get rid of them.

Importance of sex in the women's lives

The final question of the interviews (although it should be remembered that this was not the end point of my work with the women) was 'is sex important to you?'. As I was certain that they all understood the word 'important', I left each woman to interpret the question in whichever way was most meaningful for her.

Three women said that sex was important and, interestingly, two of them said that this was because of pregnancy. One of these meant it in a negative context – that is, if you accidentally got pregnant this would be an important matter.[5] The other mentioned pregnancy in a positive context – that is, that sex was important because of the potential for children and that it was, therefore, especially important for younger people like herself (she was in her thirties). When I asked if she thought older people did not have sex, she replied: 'They do but their periods stop at 45 and they can't have children after that' (TM).

5   This woman *had* got pregnant herself, aged nineteen, and although I cannot be certain it was an unplanned pregnancy, it seems likely that it would have been. Her child had been removed from her care.

Two other women said that sex was important to them but they qualified this. One said: 'It's important, but not very important, it depends on who it's with and what happens' (EY). For the other, it was a much more complex picture. She said that it was important for her boyfriend and that she was willing to do it but only until they left the hospital to move into a hostel in the community (an event that was due to take place shortly afterwards). She hoped they would be able to marry then:

MM: OK, but if you *were* married, would you want to have sex?

TC: I'll have to ask him that.

MM: What do *you* want?

TC: I would have to have sex with him if he wanted sex with me.

MM: That's a bit different. Think what *you* would like, for *yourself*, don't think about D. for the minute.

TC: I would tell him that I wouldn't want any more sex... I want to marry my boyfriend.

MM: Does he want to marry you?

TC: He does.

MM: How do you know that?

TC: I told him.

MM: I know you've told him, but what's he said to you?

TC: He hasn't said nothing to me yet. I'm going to tell him to tell himself to marry me.

Two women said that sex was sometimes important, not always, but did not elaborate. However, the majority, ten of the seventeen women, said, usually, quite simply and starkly, that sex was not important to them. Only one elaborated and this was to distinguish between sex, which she did not value, and the relationship, which she did: 'Sex is not important to me, no. But having friends is. But G. mixes the two together, he wants friendship and sex, whereas with me, I just want his friendship. But I suppose that's men, isn't it?' (KN).

What the women have had to say about their personal and sexual lives and their bodies has clearly raised many important and interesting points. The next chapter discusses the key points, integrating the findings from this study with what, if anything, the literature has to say about them.

CHAPTER FIVE

What Does It All Mean?
Analysis and Discussion

The picture that emerged from most, though not all, of the women inter-viewed for this study was a generally negative one in relation to how they felt about their sexual lives. This is also true for the much larger group of women with learning disabilities I have worked with (McCarthy 1993, 1996a, 1996b). Most women in this study, in fact, did not consider themselves to *be* sexual, despite regularly engaging in sexual activity. The reasons for this are complex but in this chapter I draw out four key factors which contribute most strongly to the women's generally negative experiences. These four factors are:

- a lack of sexual agency amongst the women themselves
- the actual sexual activity that takes place
- the fact that this is experienced on a predominantly physical level
- the very high levels of sexual abuse which the women experience.

Each of these will be discussed at some length. The purpose of this analysis is that in isolating these factors, my findings from a relatively small of group of women become generalisable to much larger numbers. If these factors are responsible for the generally negative experiences of the women in this study and if they are present in the lives of other women with learning disabilities (and, indeed, without), it is likely that those women will be experiencing their sexuality negatively too.

In the rest of this chapter I discuss other important findings, including the differences between hospital and community settings.

Lack of sexual agency

By my suggestion that there is a lack of sexual agency, I am referring to absence of the women *deciding for themselves* what they wanted to do, with whom, when and how. On the whole, it was men who made these decisions and the woman's choice was either to comply or resist. As resistance carries with it the possibility, or, in some cases, the probability, of negative sanctions for the woman, compliance is often the safer 'choice' (MacKinnon 1987). This is a traditional pattern of heterosexual behaviour for women without disabilities too: 'When women do not initiate, or initiate rarely, they also acquiesce to participating in sexual behaviours they themselves would not have chosen' (Wyatt, Newcomb and Riederle 1993, p.30). This pattern is obviously not true for all women and with the greater sexual freedoms which some women have gained in recent decades, many have increased their sense of autonomy in relation to their sexuality. However, this traditional pattern has been far from overturned, even amongst younger Western women, who might have been thought most likely to have become more assertive. The recent research from the Women Risk and AIDS Project (WRAP) and Men Risk and AIDS Project (MRAP) (see Holland *et al.* 1998 for full details) found that the majority of sexual behaviours between young men and women in Britain were male led, that a quarter of the young women had experienced 'unwanted sexual intercourse in response to pressure from men' (Holland *et al.* 1991a, p.3) and that it was 'unusual for young women to discuss sex in terms of their own pleasure, rather than men's needs' (Holland *et al.* 1991b, p.20).

Second, the lack of sexual agency is also indicated by the generally low reported level (one-third) of masturbation amongst the women interviewed in this study. This is much lower than other reported surveys involving non-disabled women – for example, 82 per cent (Hite 1976), 81 per cent (Quilliam 1994). Caution needs to be taken in making comparisons, because of the much larger sample sizes in these other studies and differences in methodology. Whether women with learning disabilities really do masturbate less than other women or whether they feel less able to say so is impossible to know. Probably, both factors are true and until women with learning disabilities feel more comfortable talking about the subject (which could possibly be achieved by sensitive sex education which encourages it and from more openness about it generally), further insights into this are unlikely to be gained.

The third way in which a lack of sexual agency is indicated for the women with learning disabilities is the apparently very low levels of sexual activity between women. No woman in this study said that she had had any sexual contact with, or sexual feelings for, another woman and this is true of the much larger group of women with learning disabilities I have worked with (with one exception). The literature contains nothing but the occasional passing reference to lesbianism, usually to the effect that sex between women seems very uncommon (McCarthy and Thompson 1998) or that 'it seems exceptionally difficult for women with learning difficulties to recognise themselves as lesbians' (Walmsley 1993, p.94). However, the possibilities (and problems) concerning lesbian sexuality for women with learning disabilities are beginning to be discussed (a recent conference on *Sexuality and Women with Learning Disabilities* convened by myself included a well-attended workshop on lesbian sexuality) and it is very important that such initiatives are sustained and developed. It seems highly unlikely that women with learning disabilities would not be attracted to other women in similar proportions to other groups of women in society. Moreover, it could be argued, as it very frequently is for men with learning disabilities (Thompson 1994a, 1994b), that their historical segregation in services would have meant that women with learning disabilities would have more opportunity than other women to form lesbian relationships. My own speculations (based on what I have learnt about the sexual behaviour of both women and men) as to why lesbian sexual activity seems to be so under-represented amongst women with learning disabilities are: that women are not socialised or accustomed to taking the initiative sexually; that women are more likely to want sex in the context of an established relationship and, with no role models or support for lesbian relationships, these are unlikely to develop; attraction to a particular individual is more likely to encourage a woman to have sex, so if a woman is not sexually attracted to another woman, she is unlikely to have sex with her (whereas men will have sex anyway, regardless of whether they 'fancy' someone or not); many women learn what sex is through abuse by men, but as they are rarely abused by women, they do not learn what sex between women is; most sex between men and women in institutions involves an exchange of sex for money and there is no history of women paying anyone for sex, therefore there is no incentive or motivation for women to engage in this.

As with women's masturbation, there is undoubtedly some element of under-reporting from women with learning disabilities about their sexual activity with other women. Once again, until the subject becomes more 'legitimate' to talk about, we are unlikely to get a clearer picture. There are now some resources which enable this legitimisation – a video resource from New Zealand (Family Planning Association, Auckland 1997) contains a story about romantic love between two women with learning disabilities, with a lesbian member of staff acting as a positive role model for the women. There are also some specialist sex education resources for people with learning disabilities which are inclusive and explicit regarding images of lesbian sexuality (McCarthy and Thompson 1998; O'Sullivan and Gillies 1993). However, others avoid explicit imagery only in the case of lesbian sex and include it for heterosexuals and gay men (West London Health Promotion Agency 1994). In the learning disability field, as with sex education in mainstream schools, the development of anti-heterosexist (and, indeed, anti-sexist and anti-racist) sex education programmes is relatively new and largely unevaluated (Thomson 1994). So, it remains to be seen whether it does have an impact on women's ability to develop confidence in a lesbian identity. However, for the sake of those people who are attracted to their own sex and for those who are not but who need to develop respect and sensitivity, it should be delivered as a matter of course.

The sexual activity

The second factor which I believe contributes to the generally negative view the women had of their sexual lives relates to what actually happens to them sexually. As indicated in the previous chapter, sex, for half the women, was exclusively, and for the other half, predominantly, penetrative sex. Over half the women who gave details (nine out of sixteen) had anal intercourse, which was rated negatively by all of them. The reasons women gave for disliking it were not related to social taboos or believing it was wrong but were prag-matic reasons – it caused them considerable physical pain. Whether women with learning disabilities experience anal intercourse more frequently than other women is impossible to know. When I have discussed my work with various professionals there is a 'gut feeling' (which I share) that it is more common amongst men and women with learning disabilities than other het-erosexuals. But this is not based on any evidence, just a 'sense' people have, possibly extrapolating from their own (lack of) experience. However, what research evidence there is shows quite a wide variation in reported rates for anal intercourse between men and women: rates (which the researchers describe as 'surprisingly high') of 20 per cent and 25 per cent for adolescents in Australia and USA have been recorded (Moore and Rosenthal 1993); rates between 20 per cent and 50 per cent for adult women in the USA are suggested (Wyatt, Newcomb and Riederle 1993); although rates for adults in Britain are considerably lower – that is, almost 14 per cent of heterosexual men and 13 per cent of women report ever having had anal intercourse (Wellings *et al.* 1994). However, these research reports give no indication of whether anal intercourse was regularly practised or whether it was tried just once. Moreover, they give no reports of whether the women like or dislike it. Quilliam's (1994) study of British women suggests that anal sex is practised by a minority of women and disliked by the majority who have tried it. The WRAP research also describes it as a minority activity that was 'particularly disliked' by women (Holland *et al.* 1993). Friday's (1991) study of women's sexual fantasies suggests that as women become more sexually confident and assertive, fantasies about anal sex increase. However, as sexual fantasy and reality rarely have much in common, this should not be taken to mean that women are increasingly trying and liking anal sex. There is simply no way of knowing this as heterosexual anal sex is a 'behaviour long neglected by research' (Wyatt, Newcomb and Riederle 1993, p.29).

The women with learning disabilities interviewed for this study, and, indeed, all the women from the wider group I have worked with over the past six or seven years, have reported that their sexual experiences with men are generally devoid of those non-penetrative activities which other women (Hite 1976; Quilliam 1994) have named as sources of pleasure – for example, kissing, caressing, skin contact, stimulation (with partner's hands and mouth) of breasts, genitals and other erogenous zones. This is not to imply that women generally do not like or want vaginal penetration and would prefer these other activities. It is not an either/or situation. Most women who have reported their sexual desires to researchers imply that they want both. What seems very clear is that few women would be satisfied with what is offered to most women with learning disabilities – that is, vaginal and/or anal penetration with little or nothing else to arouse the woman prior, during or after it (see p.142). However limited the sexual lives of women with learning disabilities appear to be, it is important to note that such experiences are not unique to them. Cross-culturally and historically, many other women have also lived their entire lives in similar ways – for example, Gordon (1990) describes how, in nineteenth-century America, women were not expected to get undressed during sex and that intercourse was usually reduced to such a quick act of penetration that the women never had time to become aroused.

There is very little other research which details how people with learning disabilities actually experience their sexual lives. That which I am familiar with confirms the findings in this research study. Andron (1983) and Andron and Ventura (1987) report from their work with married couples with learning disabilities that most of the women did not know about their clitoris, did not experience orgasm or, indeed, have any concept of what it involved and that 'sex play was basically non existent. Sex was understood as penis-vagina intercourse' (Andron and Ventura 1987, p.33).

The emphasis on the physical experience

The third factor which contributes to the women's generally negative view of their sexual lives relates to the fact that sex seems to be experienced largely, or in some cases purely, on a physical level. In the previous chapter I wrote about the psychological disengagement which some of the women seemed to experience during sex and suggested that this may be a coping strategy for the, sometimes, very unpleasant situations they found themselves in. In addition to that, there also seemed to be a lack of emotional intensity about sex for the women I interviewed. Both these factors have been noted elsewhere in the literature related to the sexual experiences of women with learning disabilities (Kiehlbauch Cruz, Price-Williams and Andron 1988) as well as men (Thompson and Brown 1998). This may be due to the fact that the women did not have a wide, or even adequate, vocabulary to describe their emotions and/or like many others they may have been too embarrassed to express their emotions to someone else. It should be emphasised that I am not saying that women with learning disabilities do not feel any emotions connected with sex. For example, my findings do not concur with those of Rees and Berchert (1992, p.144) who state that 'in training over a thousand people with mental retardation, we have never encountered a client who has mentioned that love or caring are important parts of a sexual relationship'. Indeed, half the women in this study who gave reasons why they had sex said it was because they loved or liked the men they were with. However, my contention is that engaging in sex with someone you love is not the same as giving or receiving sexual contact as an expression of that love. Although I appreciate that it would have been very difficult for the women to put into words (as, indeed, it is even for people without learning disabilities), sex as a physical communication of love or affection did not seem to be a reason why the women engaged in sex with men or how they perceived the sex they got from men. This, I believe, connects back to the ideas I first raised in Chapter

One about the social construction of sex and 'sexual scripts' (Gagnon 1977). Gagnon argues that 'people learn to become sexual in the same way they become everything else. Without much reflection, they pick up directions from their social environment. They acquire and assemble meanings, skills and values from the people around them' (p.2). Moreover, Gagnon argues that sex is only experienced as very special and emotionally charged because people have been taught to believe it *is* special. Therefore, if people have not been taught that certain things are meant to be erotic, intimate, passionate, sexy, they will not assign these meanings to them. Tiefer (1995) takes up these arguments in her provocatively entitled book *Sex Is Not A Natural Act*. She writes:

> So, if sex is not a natural act, a biological given, a human universal, what is it? I would say it's a concept, first of all – a concept with shifting, but deeply felt definitions. Conceptualising sex is a way of corralling and discussing certain human potentials for consciousness, behaviour, and expression that are available to be developed by social forces, that is available to be produced, changed, modified, organized and defined. Like Jell-O, sexuality has no shape without a container, in this case a sociohistorical container of meaning and regulation. (p.7)

As the women with learning disabilities in this study describe, their avenues for learning the meanings ascribed to sex were few in number and very narrow in the scope of the information that was imparted. Some had learned about sex from direct experience (not an unusual avenue, as the WRAP researchers found (Holland *et al.* 1998), and much of this experience was abusive. Others had learnt factual things about menstruation, reproduction and contraception. None suggested that anyone had ever informed them about their potential feelings, about pleasure, desire, arousal. Men, by having consented sex with them or by sexually abusing them, were teaching the women about sex. But, as I have demonstrated in my findings, few men, if any of them, seemed to have been concerned with the women's feelings, pleasure, desire or arousal. The question needs to be asked, then, if the women were not learning their 'sexual scripts' from sex education or from their direct experience, how else could they learn it? Informally through talking with friends is one possibility but none of the women I interviewed suggested that this happened for them. The media is another possibility, although, because of literacy problems, for most women with learning disabilities this is likely to be confined to the television. This differs for other women, who get much information from written sources, such as magazines and books (Thomson and Scott 1991). As Chapter Four shows, I did ask the women specifically what they had seen about sex on television. Only one-third of the women answered the question and none of them related what they had seen about sex on television to their own sexual experiences. Interestingly, in some cases this was because the sex on television was more passionate and intimate than their own experiences. Given that actual genital sexual activity is rarely shown on terrestrial television, what the women would have been watching was nakedness, kissing, touching and general writhing about – all the things most women reported as being absent in their own sexual activity. It is not surprising, then, that they did not relate to what they saw or learn anything useful from it that they could transfer to their own lives. It is interesting that Andron (1983) and Andron and Ventura (1987) (who, incidentally, also come to the same conclusions as I do regarding the lack of development of a psycho-sexual script) note that television is a source of useless, rather than useful, information about sex for people with learning disabilities: 'From the news, they have gained knowledge of unusual circum- stances such as babies born at 25 weeks gestation and of pregnancy in a female who had a hysterectomy, but little or no understanding of their own bodies and how they function' (Andron and Ventura 1987, p.33). I can echo this with my findings – one of the women interviewed in this study knew from television that people could have sex-change operations and that a 62-year-old post-menopausal woman had had a baby, but she had no idea that she could not get pregnant through oral sex.

My suggestion here is that if you have never learned from external sources that sex can be, and in many people's minds is *meant* to be, a significant and emotional event or process and you have not learned it from internal sources – that is, your body being aroused in such a way that it produces significant or special feelings – then sex is likely to remain on the level of the physical. And the physical experience, as most of the women were well able to describe, was generally an uncomfortable or painful one. Andron and Ventura (1987) confirm this in their work and conclude, exactly as I have, that this is due to lack of lubrication prior to penetration. However, they are only referring to vaginal intercourse as, regrettably, anal sex is not mentioned in their work.

The level and impact of sexual abuse

The fourth reason why most women had a generally negative outlook regarding sex was the fact that most of them had experienced sexual abuse of one kind or another: 14 out of 17 (82%) described at least one, and some several, act(s) of sexual abuse. This is a very high prevalence rate, much higher than reported rates for other women – for example, Hall's London study *Ask Any Woman* (1985) reported prevalence rate of 17 per cent for rape and 20 per cent for attempted rape; Russell's (1984) research in the USA reported 41 per cent of women experiencing rape or attempted rape; Randall and Haskell's study (1995) in Canada found that 56 per cent of women had experienced rape or attempted rape at some point in their childhood or adulthood, with the rate rising to two out of three women if the definition of sexual abuse was broader and encompassed all forms of unwanted sexual touch or intrusion.

Differences in sample sizes, methodologies and differences in definitions of sexual abuse make it extremely difficult to compare like with like. There are two main reasons why the prevalence rate of abuse may be so high in this study: first, a broad definition of sexual abuse was used (being made to do any kind of sex which the women had not wanted) and, second, the women in this study were not a random sample. They had been referred (in fifteen cases) or referred themselves (two cases) as being in need of, or able to benefit from, education and counselling on sexual matters. For seven women it was already known that they had possibly or definitely been sexually abused and this was part of the reason for referral. However, this means that at least half the abused women had not been referred for reasons connected to the abuse. This is a somewhat higher rate than the overall pattern of referrals to the Sex Education Team, where only 35 per cent of all abused clients were referred for that reason (McCarthy and Thompson 1997). In effect, this means that the very high prevalence rate of abuse is only partly due to the women being a selected, not random, sample. Using the same broad definition of sexual abuse, the prevalence rate for all women with learning disabilities referred to the Sex Education Team over a five-year period (in effect, the vast majority of my client group during my work in this field) was 61 per cent (McCarthy and Thompson 1997). A prevalence study which matches quite closely the methodology used in the McCarthy and Thompson study (i.e. based on discussions from people with learning disabilities themselves as well as case histories) was undertaken in the USA by Hard and Plumb (1987) (see p.70). It is interesting to see that their prevalence rate of sexual abuse for women with learning disabilities was 83 per cent. This is almost exactly the same as mine, despite the fact that the Hard and Plumb sample was much bigger, involving all the people attending a day service and not just those who had been identified as having specific needs relating to sexuality. Likewise, Stromsness' 1993 study (see p.71), based on interviews with 14 women with mild learning disabilities in the USA, found a sexual abuse prevalence rate of 79 per cent, which is, again, very similar to my findings.

Because many of the women with learning disabilities in this study had experienced some form of sexual abuse at one, or various, point(s) in their lives, this would probably have made it difficult for them to experience other sexual encounters positively and/or to frame them as such. Other research concerning non-disabled women (Kelly 1988; Orlando and Koss 1983; Wyatt, Newcomb and Riederle 1993) and disabled women (Kiehlbauch Cruz, Price-Williams and Andron 1988) suggests that abusive sexual experiences can have a negative impact on women's subsequent consented sexual experiences. It is important to try to understand what links there may be between the two different types of experiences, although this is difficult to do because, as Wyatt, Newcomb and Riederle have pointed out, 'sex research has developed as a field of research quite separate from child sexual abuse or adult rape' (1993, p.6). Wyatt and her colleagues argue for research that integrates women's experiences of both consented and abusive sex, which has been my intention in this study.

It is my contention that it is the combination of a large *quantity* of sexual abuse against the women in this study and the low *quality* of much of the consented sex they have that contributes to their generally negative view of sex. Indeed, as an outsider hearing their experiences second-hand, it was often difficult to distinguish between what was abusive and what was not. This must also have been difficult for the women themselves. Consider KN, for example, who would 'give in' to men's demands and pressure and have sex she neither liked nor wanted, to 'shut them up' and stop the pressure. Or EY who said she sometimes let men continue to have sex with her, even though it was painful, because of fears that they would hit her if she told them to stop. Or TC who was quite sure the price to be paid would be physical violence and the end of the relationship if she refused to have sex with her boyfriend. Are these acts of consented sex, pressured sex or sexual abuse? Those working with non-disabled women who experience violence and pressure in relationships with men argue clearly that a woman's ability to give free consent is compromised in these situations: 'When the female partner in the relationship knows that the other can and will hurt her, she needs to take this into account in every aspect of the relationship, not only when the threat is immediate and imminent' (Eisikovits and Buchbinder 1997, p.488).

In this study, and in my wider experience of working with women with learning disabilities (McCarthy and Thompson 1997), actual acts of physical force were sometimes, but not usually, used to subdue a woman's will and force sex upon her. But a woman's will can be progressively subdued over time and/or subsumed over seemingly more urgent needs. Men who take advantage of the women's addiction to smoking and so offer cigarettes for sex, or those who take advantage of the very socially isolated lives women in hospitals lead and offer rides in their car for sex, are exerting forms of pressure that no court of law would be interested in. Women who consent to sex in such circumstances are viewed by many as only having themselves to blame. As I explained in Chapter Four, I think it is inaccurate and unhelpful to label individual women in these situation as prostitutes or as being especially 'promiscuous', as if there were something inherently 'wrong' with them. Rather, we should examine the abnormal situations they live in and see their behaviour as a response to that (Brown 1992). Burns (1993, 1998) has described very clearly how achieving a valued identity as a woman is in itself a way of shaking off the devalued identity of a person with learning disabilities. As other valued roles for women, such as those of wife, mother/grandmother, career woman, etc, are usually denied to women with learning disabilities, embracing the role of sexual partner to a man, especially a more intellectually able man, is the only positive choice open to some women. If being exploited, oppressed or even abused is the price to be paid, that is a worthwhile trade-off in the eyes of many women with learning disabilities (Stromsness 1993).

Much of the learning disability literature on consent to sexual activity (see, for example, Kaeser 1992) focuses on assessing an individual's ability to give consent and the conditions which need to be in place – that is, *capacity* (the aptitude to acquire knowledge); the person needs to be *informed* (understand the advantages and disadvantages of a decision); *voluntariness* (absence of coercion, force or duress) (Ames 1991). Such approaches look at individuals at specific moments of time and not at the overall social context in which they are placed. Little attention is paid to feminist theories about the inherent difficulties regarding relationships which are fundamentally unequal to start with when those inequalities are based predominantly on gender (see Brown and Turk 1992 for an exception).

In my view, this lack of feminist perspective within the wider learning disability field is a significant weakness. When we pay careful attention to what women with learning disabilities say about their sexual lives, it becomes clear that in many cases the women's ability to give free and informed consent to sex has been compromised by some particular factors which have to do with their learning disability, but, importantly, also some particular factors which have to do with their being women:

> When sex is violent, women may have lost control over what is done to us, but the absence of force does not ensure the presence of that control. Nor, under conditions of male dominance, does the presence of force make an interaction nonsexual. If sex is normally something men do to women, the issue is less whether there was force and more whether consent is a meaningful concept. (MacKinnon 1987, p.144)

This echoes Pateman's (1980) earlier work on consent, in which she discusses women's consent to sex in the wider context of 'consent theory'. Pateman argues that unless there is genuine freedom and equality between women and men, 'an egalitarian sexual relationship...cannot be grounded in consent' (p.164). Pateman also asserts that: 'Consent as an ideology cannot be distinguished from habitual acquiescence, assent, silent dissent, submission, or even enforced submission. Unless refusal of consent or withdrawal of consent are real possibilities, we can no longer speak of "consent" in any genuine sense' (p.150).

Some of the women in this research, and, indeed, in that of others (e.g. Gavey 1992; Holland *et al.* 1991a, 1991b), have shown that being able to *not* consent is far from straightforward. Gavey's work illustrates how the stark options of consent or non-consent are simply not perceived as distinct choices by some women. Thus the apparent or actual complicity of some women with what men want from them sexually is a highly complex process which is influenced by many different discourses regarding heterosexuality. Gavey looks at a number of these discourses which lead women to engage in unwanted sex with men, including what is perceived to be 'normal' heterosexual behaviour – women having sex with men as a way of taking care of them – or for pragmatic reasons – such as avoiding arguments or wanting to get to sleep. Her research also highlights what she calls the 'ultimate pragmatic reason' – that is, 'consenting' to sex to avoid being raped.

The law, as it has traditionally been allowed to interpret women's consent (or lack thereof), is also highly problematic. Pateman (1980) points out that:

> ...a woman's explicit 'no' is all too frequently disregarded or reinterpreted as 'consent'. However, if 'no', when uttered by a woman, is to be reinterpreted as 'yes', then all the comfortable assumptions about her 'consent' are also thrown into disarray. Why should a woman's 'yes' be more privileged, be any less open to invalidation, than her 'no'? (p.162)

However, the law, as it is applied, and the dominant discourses of heterosexuality it feeds from often turn out to mean that if a woman says yes, she means yes. If she says no, she means yes. And if she says nothing at all, she means yes. This position is absurd and outdated and, in recognition of this, Lees (1996) has called for a move away from the simplistic concept of consent, towards a more 'modern communicative model of sexuality' (p.260).

It is impossible to unpack the different strands of oppression and to know whether the high levels of sexual abuse of women with learning disabilities and the lack of response to it by learning disability services or the law is *primarily* because they are women or because they have learning disabilities. However, what we can do is observe that many women with learning disabilities often decide not to report sexual abuse because they know, instinctively or from past experience, that they would not be believed (Brown 1996; Hard and Plumb 1987) and they feel they may be blamed. In this respect they have much in common with other women who have experienced sexual abuse (Kelly 1988). One woman in this study, who lived in a community learning disability service, did not tell the staff that she was being pestered by a man for sex because she thought the staff would think badly of her. Another lived in a hospital which had a tunnel under the road which ran through the two sites of the hospital. Many women were anxious about using the tunnel, especially at night. I personally avoided it in the dark and used the road instead. But hospital residents were encouraged to use it so that they did not risk a road accident. One woman had been touched in a sexual way by a male resident in the tunnel. She had neither invited nor liked the touch but did not report the incident to the staff. When I asked what she thought the staff would say if she did report it, her immediate reply was 'They'd say "why were you in the tunnel?"' (GJ). One can only presume that if she had been knocked over crossing the road, she would have been asked 'why weren't you in the tunnel?' There is also evidence that there is a greater readiness to believe and respond to the sexual abuse of men with learning disabilities compared to their female peers: Hard and Plumb (1987) found that all men in their study were believed when they disclosed abuse, whilst 55 per cent of women were not believed. In the McCarthy and Thompson prevalence study (1997) men with learning disabilities were significantly more likely than women to have their abuse responded to in a serious fashion (i.e. by senior managers investigating or a thorough police investigation). The likely reason for these differences in responding to the sexual abuse of men and women is 'the perceived normality of heterosexual sex (including abusive sex) compared to any homosexual contact' (McCarthy and Thompson 1997, p.117).

The findings in this research study and other related work (e.g. McCarthy and Thompson 1997; Thompson 1997) indicate that there are rarely any negative sanctions for the perpetrators of sexual abuse against women with learning disabilities, especially when the perpetrators have learning disabilities themselves. When the women do report abuse, they are rarely offered specialist support, legal justice or compensation (Brown 1996). These facts also make it difficult for the women with learning disabilities (and others) to see what 'counts' as sexual abuse and what does not. It is hard to escape the conclusion that not much does 'count' as abuse and this may be one reason why the women put up with so much negative sexual attention and activity.

The positive side

It would be wrong to concentrate only on the negative side of the women's sexual lives without also drawing attention to the more positive aspects. Three of the women in this study were generally positive about their sexual lives. Only one talked in any detail about why this was – she had a boyfriend who was roughly the same age and of the same ability level as her; they lived similar lives, going to college and socialising with friends; they had a lot in common and she considered them to be equal partners in the relationship. She had been raped by two different men in the past (one her father) but felt a determination not to accept bad treatment now. She described herself as being assertive with her boyfriend and, although it was he who always took the initiative sexually and who decided what was going to happen, she felt well able to say what she did and did not want. She expressed confidence in his respectful responses to her needs – for instance, when asked what she would expect her boyfriend to do if she told him she did not like a particular sexual act, she replied in a very clear voice 'I *know* what he would do, he would stop' (DO).

Those women with long-term boyfriends valued their relationships very highly and wanted them to continue (see also Stromsness 1993). This is very important to note because, although the sex was largely unsatisfactory for the women, sex is only one part of a relationship. Moreover, as was stated in Chapter One, actually having sex does not usually take up a great deal of most people's time. Sex, therefore, can be relatively unimportant within the overall context of a relationship and this did, indeed, seem to be the case for many of the women with learning disabilities in this study and in my wider experience. Although there is much similarity between my work and that of Andron and Ventura (1987), I come to quite the opposite conclusion about the primacy of sex within the women's relationships. Andron and Ventura conclude that couples with learning disabilities often have little privacy and many of their practical needs (such as shopping, cooking, laundry, etc) are met by carers and that, therefore, 'their "couplehood" is expressed only in bed. This places a large emphasis on sex and makes the smallest problem appear a major dysfunction' (p.34). From what I learned from women with learning disabilities, 'couplehood' is not necessarily expressed through *doing* things together that couples might expect to do but, rather, through *being* together in an acknowledged relationship. And far from sex having a very big importance, the women in this study totally refute that. It has, as they clearly indicated, generally little importance in their lives and, although it may sound strange, I think this is one of the positive features to emerge from this study. This is because, although the women generally did not rate sex highly, they did not let this depress them unduly. They coped with it by not according it much importance in their lives. The development and maintenance of relationships with men were far more important to them, it seemed. Other relationships were also important – some women had friendships with other women which they valued; some were very fond of, and felt close to, particular members of staff; some women had very positive family ties, particularly with parents, which were highly valued. Coping strategies have been defined as 'any thought or action which succeeds in eliminating or ameliorating threat to the self...whether it is consciously recognised as intentional or not' (Breakwell 1986, p.79). Therefore, it seems that coping with a negative feature of one's life by relegating it to the realms of the unimportant could be seen as part of the women's resistance to, and survival from, the various negative sexual experiences.

The resistance to, and recovery from, sexual abuse by women with learning disabilities is another positive feature to emerge from this work and has been noted elsewhere in the literature (Millard 1994). Many of the women had experienced acts of abuse which could very easily have been utterly devastating to their sense of self. I am not implying that the women in this study were not damaged by their abuse at all. On the contrary, some had mental health problems, including depression and panic attacks, and others had self-injurious and challenging behaviour. But, nevertheless, without the benefit of much, if any, therapeutic help, none of the women was incapacitated by what had happened to them. That said, there was one woman in this study who, by her own acknowledgement, would probably have done a lot more with her life had she not been raped by her father and given birth to his child. Generally speaking, however, the personal strength and resilience shown by the women in coming to terms with what happened to them and, in some cases, with what was continuing to happen, was to their great credit. It is all the more noteworthy because other research evidence indicates that women with the least internal or external resources to draw on, such as older women, poor women, women who had experienced a major life stress before the abuse, generally have more difficulty coping than others (Kelly 1988).

Another positive feature to emerge is that some of the sexual taboos which still operate to make people feel embarrassed and ashamed about sex did not seem to have a great impact on the women in this study. Regarding anal intercourse, for example, only one woman held a belief that this was morally wrong and to be avoided for that reason. None of the other women seemed to differentiate (on moral grounds) between vaginal and anal sex, nor have any awareness that these two activities are generally valued differently in society. It is interesting to note, however, that many did view oral sex as still a taboo subject. This is a reversal of the trend in the general population – women's magazines (see, for example, Meade 1993) carry explicit articles about oral sex, as do those aimed specifically at teenagers and young women. Indeed, what appears in these publications could be seen as positive encouragement for young women to engage in this particular sexual activity. To verify my assumptions about this, in September 1998 I bought the first young women's magazine that came to hand in a local newsagent (it happened to be *Eva* – 'For the girl who wants it all'). On page 45 readers were told that a 'blow-job has to be one of your boyfriend's best friends' and on page 51 a telephone advice line was advertised if 'you simply want to perfect your blow-job technique'. Various other specific sexual activities were mentioned throughout the magazine but there was no mention of anal intercourse and, indeed, this does seem to very rare – that is, there is effectively no public discourse on heterosexual anal sex (see p.206).

Also, as I indicated in Chapter Four, most of the women who had had a sexually transmitted disease or other genito-urinary infection did not seem embarrassed or ashamed of this. Although the women generally held prejudicial views regarding masturbation and lesbian sexuality, the only social taboo regarding sex with men which had a strong impact on all the women was that relating to sexual activity during menstruation. As well as practical reasons for wanting to avoid it, there was a strong sense of moral disapproval about this. It is hard to know why some sexual taboos had an impact and others did not. I can only speculate that because of the paucity of information the women had been given about sexual matters and the fact that much of it had revolved around fears of reproduction, the women may, for example, simply not have been told or 'warned' about anal sex or sexually transmitted diseases. Conversely, many of them said that they had been told about periods, often by their mothers, and it is not hard to imagine that this may have included the message 'not to let men touch you when you've got your period'.

As well as reversal of some taboos, and a significant difference in the relative frequency of certain kinds of sexual activities (see p.206), there is also a reversal in societal attitudes about whether or not engagement in sex is acceptable in the first place. Despite having worked in this field for several years, I have never heard anyone suggest that the complete abstention from sex, or going for long periods of time without a sexual partner, is in any way socially unacceptable for a person with learning disability. Taking it for granted that many adults with learning disabilities are not sexually active is a remnant of past attitudes which suggested that they were asexual. However, lack of engagement in sexual activity is not all taken for granted in other, non-disabled people, at least during their young and middle adulthood. Unlike most women with learning disabilities, many other women who either make a deliberate choice to be celibate (Cline 1993) or who simply do not have a sexual partner for prolonged periods (Bickerton 1983) feel themselves to be at the mercy of other people's judgements and, indeed, their pity. Whichever way it is experienced – that is, it can be painful if it is not wanted or misunderstood when it is wanted – not engaging in sex is problematic for many adults and this is simply not recognised as a relevant issue for the vast majority of people with learning disabilities, especially women.

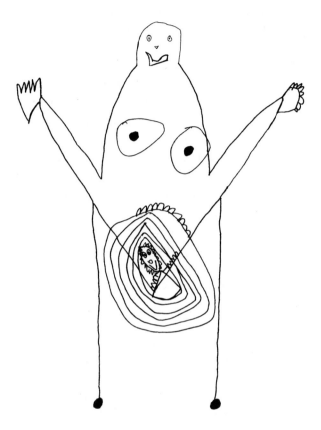

Figure 5.1

The final positive feature to mention relates to the women's desires to have children. Only three of the seventeen had had children and none had raised their children in the long term – two had their children taken into care and one had her son raised as her brother (indeed, he was both, as the woman's own father was the child's father). Some of the women expressed no wish to have a child, others did. All seemed very aware that other people, particularly staff, did not think motherhood was a realistic option for people like them. This has been noted elsewhere in the literature: 'People like us don't have babies. No one at the centre does apart from staff. Some people have their stomachs taken out' (Woman with learning disabilities quoted in Atkinson and Williams 1990, p.175). Despite this, seven of the seventeen women actively resisted this notion, stating clearly and on more than one occasion, that they wanted children, they liked children, they felt they could cope with looking after them and that their lives were lacking something without them. The fact that most, if not all, were unlikely to realise their ambitions should not be taken as signs of passive acceptance. The women wanted children despite the ideologies which had them labelled as unfit parents before they even began (Booth and Booth 1994) and despite their own limitations, which probably would have meant the stresses of childcare would have been beyond what they could cope with.

It was interesting to note that two women in this study believed that they would be able to adopt children if they wanted to. Although this was not a commonly expressed belief, it has been mentioned to me before by other women with learning disabilities I have worked with. It is hard to imagine that they would ever have been seriously advised that this may be a possibility for them but I think that they may have picked up the common, if somewhat old-fashioned, understanding of adoption as an option for 'people who can't have their own children' and applied it to themselves.

Body image

In common with many other women (Brownmiller 1986), most women with learning disabilities in this study found it very difficult to say anything positive about their bodies. It was hard to tell whether the difficulty was in *believing* that there was anything positive about their bodies or in actually *saying* positive things. I suspect it was primarily the former because a negative body image is generally acknowledged to be one of the most acutely felt forms of oppression for women (Wolf 1990). That women with learning disabilities respond to this oppression in similar ways to other women was confirmed by the fact that ten of the women were dissatisfied with the same thing, namely their weight. As only one of these ten women would have been considered by most people to be 'genuinely' overweight (as opposed to on the plump or heavy side), the women had clearly internalised society's high expectations regarding how slim women should be. The women reported that staff in learning disability services directly encouraged them to lose weight and that staff and peers complimented them when they were thin.

I am not suggesting here that the weight of people with learning disabilities should never be the concern of staff. Some people, particularly those with additional physical disabilities that may make eating difficult, may well be very underweight. Conversely, there are some conditions, such as Down's Syndrome, which may predispose people to being overweight

(Bell and Bhate 1992). All too often, however, being 'overweight' is equated with assumptions of being unfit or unhealthy, when neither may be the case. Seventy-seven per cent of the learning disability services in a recent study indicated that encouraging weight loss was the key indicator of their attempts at a healthy lifestyle initiative for their service users (Turner 1996). Turner does not report (nor have I seen any attention paid to this in services) as to how people with learning disabilities, especially women, may actually *feel* about their weight. My findings would indicate that most women with learning disabilities would welcome initiatives aimed at helping them lose weight. Nevertheless, consideration needs to be given to supporting individuals to resist these pressures if they want to, otherwise learning disability services will be perpetuating unrealistic and unfair expectations on women. The politics, as well as the pleasures, of weight loss for women need to be considered (Brown 1996).

I regret that I did not discuss the matter of body hair and facial hair with the women in this study as it seems very likely that these would also have been vexed issues (see McCarthy 1998a for a fuller discussion on this). On other occasions when I have talked to women with learning disabilities about this, those whose body hair is left to grow have indicated that they do not like this but accept that they have to live with it because they cannot remove it themselves and other people do not consider it important to do so. It has seemed to be something which they recognise sets them apart from other, non-disabled women, who they rarely, if ever, see with body/facial hair. When women with learning disabilities internalise their devalued status both as women and as people with a disability (Downes 1982), it should not be surprising that so few have positive images of themselves.

Contraception

My findings that all the women in this study used, or had used, only three methods of contraception – the Pill, Depo-Provera, Intra-Uterine Devices (IUDs) – reflects my wider experience of working with women with learning disabilities. The literature also confirms that these three methods are the only ones used by most women with learning disabilities, with barrier methods being reported as unheard of (Chamberlain *et al.* 1984). It is no coincidence that the three methods commonly used are those which require little or no 'active user participation' (Chamberlain *et al.* 1984, p.449). The reliance on low/no maintenance methods assumes that women with learning disabilities are incapable or unreliable when it comes to managing their own fertility. It is undeniably the case that some women with learning disabilities would find making decisions about which type of contraception to use very difficult and would also find it hard or impossible to manage the practicalities of some methods. However, it is also undeniable that many women with learning disabilities, including those in this study, are not given sufficient or appropriate information and support to make those choices themselves. As Williams (1992) states, 'The imposition of contraception, like the long-lasting drug Depo-Provera…reveals pressures to discourage the fertility of certain groups of women' (p.156). Certainly, Depo-Provera is disproportionately used with women with learning disabilities. What little literature there is on the topic (e.g. Chamberlain *et al.* 1984; Elkins 1994) suggests that it is generally well tolerated with minimal side effects, but neither study reports any views of women with learning disabilities themselves.

IUDs are not generally the contraception of choice of younger women who have not had any children, yet they are frequently used for women with learning disabilities in these categories (Chamberlain *et al.* 1984; Elkins 1994). (Incidentally, the Chamberlain study is entitled *Issues in Fertility Control for Mentally Retarded Adolescents,* yet actually relates to girls and women aged 11–23, a curiously broad definition of adolescence.) Despite the common side-effect of heavy bleeding during menstruation (see below for discussion), the relative popularity of the IUD for women with learning disabilities seems to be due to the fact that it requires little maintenance – once inserted, it can be 'forgotten'. In my experience working with women with learning disabilities, IUDs can be literally forgotten by all concerned, with no one checking or replacing them for years on end. Sometimes, the woman herself (as with FM in this study) can forget she has one *in situ.*

The lack of use of barrier methods of contraception amongst women with learning disabilities is interesting. Use of condoms is mentioned widely in the literature but this is almost exclusively in relation to HIV prevention. Use of the cap or diaphragm is almost entirely overlooked (see the video *Between Ourselves* (1988) for a notable exception). Overlooking the use of the cap is regrettable because some women like this method because of the sense of control it gives them over their own fertility (Phillips and Rakusen 1989). However, for women with learning disabilities it is generally assumed that they would be incapable of managing it reliably. Despite my implied criticism here, the very real practicalities of using the cap should not be dismissed: a woman has to be willing to touch her genitals; it is tricky to learn how to insert it properly; a woman has to remember to insert and remove it at the right times; and as many women with learning disabilities do not have sex in their bedrooms, they would have to remember to carry it around with them. The hurried nature of much of the sexual activity women with learning disabilities have reported to me suggests that caps *would* be impractical. Use of the female condom is also likely to be very limited amongst women with learning disabilities for the same reasons (McCarthy and Thompson 1998).

This study did not specifically focus on other matters related to women's sexual and reproductive health, such as breast and cervical screening or the

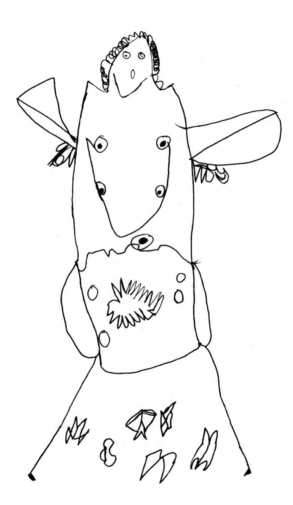

Figure 5.2 'Hormones give you hassle'

menopause. These remain very much under-researched areas (Brown 1996) and some recent research which has appeared is shocking in its disregard for the rights of women with learning disabilities to be treated as other women. Huovinen (1996), for example, describes the positive effects of therapeutic amenorrhea (the deliberate stopping of periods) for women with learning disabilities as being 'so obvious' that they do not merit discussion. He conducted a research study in Finland to see at what point this medical intervention should stop, because it is obviously unnecessary after the menopause. His conclusion was 'even in mentally retarded women menopause is individual' (p.61). It beggars belief that anyone might have thought that all women with learning disabilities would reach menopause at the same time and one cannot help but be concerned that Finnish taxpayers' money is funding such research.

The reason for prescribing contraception to women with learning disabilities is not always a straightforward matter of preventing an unwanted pregnancy in a sexually active woman of childbearing age. Many times when I have questioned why a woman with learning disabilities who was not sexually active was on the Pill I have been told by staff and carers that it is because of heavy or painful periods (McCarthy and Thompson 1992). Whilst not dismissing these as genuine concerns, I must say that it does seem to be a *very* common problem for women with learning disabilities, to the point where I cannot help wondering whether staff and carers are not exaggerating it in order to justify being able to use the Pill or, indeed, other methods of contraception, as a long-term strategy to avoid any possibility of pregnancy for the whole of a woman's reproductive life. The very-long term use of the Pill and the ways in which IUDs and Depo-Provera are used with women with learning disabilities, combined with a lack of attention to side-effects and after-effects, suggests that less importance is placed on their health and future fertility than on other women's.

Other reasons why contraception is given to control or eliminate menstruation, particularly amongst women with more severe disabilities, is that they would be unable to practically manage their periods and/or that they would be very distressed or confused by the sight of blood (Taylor and Carlson 1993). There is little research evidence to substantiate this. However, there *is* evidence that attitudes towards menstruation vary widely amongst women and, particularly, between women and men, with men generally holding more negative and oppressive attitudes (Laws 1990). As the medical profession is male dominated, this may partly explain why contraception is so readily prescribed for reasons other than preventing unwanted pregnancies.

It is undoubtedly the case that, just as for many other women, some women with learning disabilities enjoy a greater degree of personal freedom if they are using reliable contraception than might otherwise be the case (see p.56 for my argument that the availability of contraception to people with learning disabilities was one of the factors that led to a less restrictive care regime). However, the downside of this (which was certainly relevant to many of the women I have worked with, although not many in this particular study) relates to risks of sexual abuse. I have written elsewhere about the false sense of security given when women are given contraception as 'protection from the sexually active men around them' (McCarthy and Thompson 1992, p.70). Taylor and Carlson (1993) go further and point out, rightly in my view, that prescribing contraception to a woman with learning disabilities thought to be at risk of sexual abuse in fact increases her vulnerability to abuse. As much abuse is perpetrated by male family and staff members, these men would presumably know that as detection through pregnancy will not occur, their chances of being caught and identified are reduced.

Hospital and community settings

When I first began my work in this field I expected to find fundamentally different patterns of sexual behaviour and experiences depending on whether people with learning disabilities lived in hospital or community settings. This expectation was reflected in the title of the thesis I wrote for my doctorate ('The sexual experiences and sexual abuse of women with learning disabilities in institutional and community settings'). I expected the situations of individuals to be significantly worse in hospitals, due primarily to a lack of privacy but also to the general dehumanising effects of institutions.

One of the disappointing findings of my work, and that of my colleagues, which is reflected in this research, is that the differences are not nearly as pronounced as I had imagined. As I outlined in Chapter Four, there were only two areas where there were clear divisions between women based in the hospital and those in the community. These differences related to the exchange of sex for money or other material rewards (with all the hospital-based but none of the community-based women engaging in this) and to the places where people conducted their sexual activity (with all the hospital-based women having to have sex in semi-private places, often in outdoor locations, whilst all the community-based women had sex in their own, or their partner's, bedroom).

The greater privacy available to the women in the community may have accounted for some other, but less stark, differences. However, because the numbers are so small, it is very difficult to make valid comparisons between the hospital- and community-based groups. Therefore, the following information is presented with caution. Access to greater privacy may have led to the fact that the three women who were most positive about their sexual experiences had all lived in community settings (although two were in hospital at the time of the interviews). Gavey's (1992) research also suggests that where opportunities for sex are constrained by lack of privacy and/or time, women tend to be dissatisfied by the experience. Greater privacy may also have affected the way women felt about engaging in masturbation, where four of the five women who said they did masturbate or had done so were in community settings.

Having greater numbers of sexual partners did seem to be associated with being in hospital. This may be partly due to the easy availability of sexual partners when very large numbers of people are congregated together. It is also likely to be partly due to the fact that institutional settings are generally not considered to be conducive to the maintenance of long-term relationships (Crossmaker 1991). However, it should be noted that four of the hospital-based women in this study had sustained very long-term relationships (i.e. lasting several years) with men.

There were some differences in the types of sexual activity the women engaged in (bearing in mind the relatively small numbers). There was a strong association between being in hospital and engaging in anal intercourse, with all eight hospital-based women having experienced it compared to only one community-based woman and one who had lived in both settings (it was not clear where she had experienced it). There was also an association (although not as strong) between a woman giving oral sex to a man and being in hospital. One reason for these differences could be a greater reluctance on the part of community-based women to speak about these more 'taboo' sexual activities, although this is speculation and I do not have any evidence to substantiate this. Another, perhaps more likely reason, is that for both groups it was the men who controlled what sexual activity took place. The women who were long-term hospital residents were largely having sex with men who were also long-term hospital residents. It is likely that many of these men would have had considerable experience of sex with other men (Thompson 1994) and may have been replicating some of their same-sex experience with women.

Lack of information about, and experience of, clitoral stimulation and orgasm was universal across both hospital- and community-based women. The only difference was that the three women who used or recognised the word 'coming' (but who, as I explained on p.137, did not really know what it meant) were all in the community settings. They were also amongst the most intellectually able and had had sex largely with men similar to, or more able than, themselves, so it is not surprising that their vocabulary for sexual matters included this term. An interesting observation is that despite the relatively high ability level of the women in this study, very few used colloquial or slang terms for sexual activities or body parts, apart from ones which are in very common usage, such as 'bum'. Apart from the one or two most able women in community settings who did occasionally use terms such as 'coming' or 'wank', there were a few other women who used words like 'fuck' or 'fucking', but this was in the context of swearing in general conversation, not to refer to sex. Men with learning disabilities have been noted as using more slang terms for sex than women of similar ability levels (McCarthy 1991). The implication of this is that sex education materials aimed directly at people with learning disabilities which use slang terms (e.g. Cambridge 1995) may be meeting the needs of men more than women.

In relation to opportunities to learn or talk about sex, there did appear to be some slight differences between women in hospital and community settings – of the five women who said that they felt that staff did not really want to discuss matters of a sexual nature, four were in hospital; of the five who said that they had had some formal sex education, four were in the community.

With regard to their feelings about their bodies and their appearance, there were some slight differences – the women in the community seemed generally less happy with their body image and appearance than the women in hospital. This could be because outside of the hospital environment the women are exposed to more societal pressures to be attractive. However, the women in hospital do watch television, see magazines and go out so this is a somewhat tenuous argument. It could be more the case that by living more ordinary lives in the community, the women have picked up inhibitions which discourage them saying positive things about themselves.

There were also some slight differences with regard to having had a sexually transmitted disease or other genito-urinary infection – the hospital-based women were more likely to have experienced these than the women in community settings. With regard to the sexually transmitted infections, this may be accounted for by the fact that the hospital-based women tended to have more sexual partners and more anal intercourse; with regard to the non-sexually transmitted genito-urinary conditions, I do not know why these would appear to be more common in the hospital-based group. I can only imagine that being surrounded by nurses and doctors, the women in hospital may have been more readily diagnosed than women living in the community.

Conclusion

Generally speaking, with regard to important factors such as control, sexual pleasure and freedom from pain and/or coercion, the overall situation was slightly better for women in community settings. However, as I have explained, the differences were not pronounced and this situation is depressing in that it is not possible to 'blame' most of the negative features of women's sexual experiences on the adverse effects of institutionalisation, as I had once naïvely expected to be able to do. The general lack of significant difference in sexual experiences for women with learning disabilities, regardless of where they are living, has largely been completely overlooked in the literature to date, with the exception of my own observations (McCarthy 1994). Anecdotally, I am aware of some professionals in the field of sexuality and learning disability who believe that there *are* significant differences and that the situation for women in terms of their sexual experiences is much better in the community than in hospital and they have criticised my work for not drawing more attention to this. However, I have not seen evidence of this. Indeed, if one compares the findings of work based entirely in community settings (e.g. Andron and Ventura 1987; Millard 1994) with those based predominantly in hospitals (e.g. McCarthy 1993) and with this study, another conclusion must be drawn: that whilst the physical environment has some impact (with all the effects of hospital environments being in the negative direction), the quality of women's sexual experiences is more directly determined by factors such as the nature of relationships between women and men, abuse and aggression from men, assertiveness from women, women's perceptions of themselves as sexual beings entitled to personal fulfilment and the existence of sex education and support in its broadest sense.

It is these factors and others which will be discussed further in the final chapter.

CHAPTER SIX

The Way Forward

Policy and Practice Recommendations

In this final chapter I will make recommendations with regard to both policy and practice issues; some in relation to learning disability services in a broad sense but, most specifically, in relation to sexuality and sexual abuse. However, before I outline my recommendations I would like to note that I am mindful of the ethical issues involved in doing so. As Holland and Ramazanoglu (1994) have pointed out, 'The issue of whose knowledge is produced from interviews, and to what ends it should be put, is particularly salient in the case of feminist research' (p.141). Like other feminist researchers, I have tried to give voice to the experiences of women who rarely have an opportunity to 'have their say'. But I have also analysed and put my own interpretations on the women's experiences. Holland and Ramazanoglu go on to say:

> Drawing policies from confused and contested meanings can never be an orderly or value-free process. Feminism plays methodological, moral and political roles in struggling to ensure that as much of women's experience as possible can be grasped, and that appropriate policy recommendations can be drawn from this experience. (p.143)

In view of this, and to minimise the chances that I may have misunderstood or misinterpreted what the women in this study have said, the following recommendations have developed primarily from the findings of this particular study but are also rooted in my broader experience in working on sexuality issues in learning disability services. They are not in order of priority.

Policy recommendations

Continuation of hospital closures

The first recommendation relates to the very broad issue of deinstitutionalisation and the provision of services in the community. Although the hospital closure policy has been fully implemented in some parts of the country, in others it has not and, at the end of the twentieth century, large hospitals for people with learning disabilities do still exist. Indeed, at the time of writing, two of the four hospitals represented in this study are still open, although one is in the last stages of closing down. As I outlined in Chapter Two, some writers are drawing attention to what they see as a process of reinstitutionalisation, with new services being developed on old hospital sites. The implications of continued hospitalisation for the sexual lives of women with learning disabilities are serious. Although this study found relatively few stark differences between the experiences of women in hospital and those in the community, those it did find were to the detriment of the women in hospitals. In addition, there is the fact that, contrary to what a lot of people think (see, for example, Marchant 1993b), hospitals can be very sexualized environments, more so than many community service settings. As I have remarked elsewhere: 'It should be obvious that living in a large hospital which has spacious grounds, with scores of other people with learning difficulties, accords more opportunities for sex than living in a small house with a few other people and higher levels of supervision' (McCarthy and Thompson 1995, p.278).

A number of women with learning disabilities who have lived in both hospital and community settings have confirmed the view that more sex happens in hospital. In this study this was most clearly expressed by the woman who said that, in relation to being in hospital, 'Sex life is different here. At home it was more now and again, not all the time like it is here' (TM).

To focus on the *amount*, rather than the *nature*, of sexual activity taking place in one setting as opposed to another may seem puzzling. However, the fact that higher levels of sexual activity are taking place in the physical environments least suited to it is a cause for concern and a policy issue. The provision of privacy for people with learning disabilities to express themselves sexually should be more of a priority for all service providers than it hitherto has been. It has long been recognised that 'where there is no privacy, there is no appropriate sexuality' (Hingsburger 1987, p.44). This impacts more on women with learning disabilities than men because, as this study illustrates, when there is little or no privacy, little time is spent on sex and sexual expression is reduced (largely at the instigation of men) down to the bare minimum of a quick engagement in sexual intercourse, which many women express dissatisfaction with. Until services grasp the nettle and prioritise the provision of private and dignified space for people with learning disabilities to have sex in, it is important that my work, and that of others (e.g. Hingsburger 1987; Thompson 1994a), continues to confront policy makers with the inevitable consequences of the lack of privacy: 'When clients talk about "having sex" it is tempting to translate this into our own culture's understanding of that – which is naked and in bed, but it is important to remember that these clients had a different experience and learnt different sexual practices' (Hingsburger 1987, p.44).

For many people with learning disabilities in hospitals and some community settings, including the women in this study, this is true. Many have never had sex in a bed and many never remove all or even most of their clothes. A lack of privacy not only reduces sex to being something rather furtive, which in itself can lead to the emotional/psychological disengagement with it I earlier outlined (see also Heyman and Huckle 1995), but it also has implications for the sexual health of people with learning disabilities. I would maintain now, just as strongly as I did some years ago, that 'it is completely unrealistic to expect people with learning difficulties to engage in safer sex activities which involve the sensual and sexual exploration of each other's bodies' (McCarthy and Thompson 1992, p.63) whilst they have little privacy. The issues for women are even more poignant: whilst they are obliged to conduct their sexual lives in undignified surroundings, they cannot be expected to develop the self-esteem that is necessary if they are to become assertive enough to negotiate sexual matters with men.

Policies to reduce risks of sexual abuse against women in learning disability services

Whilst changes at policy level will never be able to eradicate all sexual abuse in services, there is, nevertheless, much that could be done to reduce the chances of it happening. With my colleague and co-author, David Thompson, I have outlined in some detail how this might be achieved (McCarthy and Thompson 1996). I will summarise some of the key points here as the findings from this research study confirm previous impressions and arguments.

First, there needs to be concern about placing men with very mild or only borderline learning disabilities who have committed sexual offences in the remaining learning disability hospitals. There is a long history of using learning disability services as a diversion from the prison system for such men, which goes back at least as far as the 1913 Mental Deficiency Act. Various factors now contribute to the policy of placing individuals who pose a sexual risk to others in learning disability services: the Reed Committee Report (Dept. of Health and Home Office 1992) listed, amongst others, the lack of specialist provision for offenders with borderline or mild learning disabilities (p.49), many of whom, the report recognised, were sexual offenders (p.50); and the inadequate provision of medium secure units for people with learning disabilities (p.49).

In addition to this, it is quite clear to anyone familiar with learning disability hospitals today that as well as sex offenders with very mild learning disabilities, men with histories of sex offending with no learning disability in the generally accepted sense of the term are also being admitted (McCarthy and Thompson 1997; Thompson 1997). The well-publicised escape (during a visit to Chessington World of Adventure few years ago) of convicted child sex offender Trevor Holland is a case in point (see, for example, Fleet and Johnston 1996). The impact on the lives and sexual experiences of women with learning disabilities of the policy of receiving such men into learning disability services is illustrated by this research study – out of a relatively small group of nine women who had ever lived in hospitals, two had boyfriends with little or no learning disabilities who were convicted rapists.

Men who have little or no learning disability immediately gain a very high status within services, precisely because they are so much more able than the vast majority of other clients. This high status, combined with the other advantages which often go with a higher intellectual ability (such as more social skills, a history of having lived independently), make the men seem attractive to many of the women in learning disability services. However, forming sexual relationships with these men can make the women very vulnerable – not only are the women more likely than not to already have experienced sexual abuse with all the damage to confidence and self-esteem that often entails but, as sex offenders, the men have, by definition, already proved themselves to be willing and able to disregard another person's sexual rights, feelings and wishes. In addition, because of confidentiality policies, the women are not told of the men's histories of sexual offending, so are in a poor position to protect themselves. This is a very undesirable set of circumstances and one which policy makers urgently need to rectify.

The second factor which increases the vulnerability of women with learning disabilities to sexual abuse within services is the siting of Regional Secure Units (RSU) or similar services within the grounds of learning disability hospitals. In my experience of working in a hospital with such a unit on site, it was clear that men from the RSU were disproportionately named by women as the perpetrators of sexual abuse and/or physical violence; as rough and insensitive sexual partners; and as the perpetrators of sexual harassment. This study confirms that – of the six women who lived in a hospital with an RSU on site, five reported sexual and/or physical abuse by men from what was (in comparison to the rest of the hospital) a very small unit.

Third, having only mixed-sex residential accommodation is a policy decision which needs reviewing because of the potential for it to impact negatively on women with learning disabilities. As I explained in Chapter Two, it is increasingly being recognised that the biggest single group of perpetrators of sexual abuse against people with learning disabilities is, in fact, men with learning disabilities (Brown, Turk and Stein 1995; McCarthy and Thompson 1997). Ensuring that women with learning disabilities did not have to share a service with their male peers would, therefore, significantly increase their sexual safety, just as it would in mental health services (Copperman and Burrows 1992). This is something that some women with learning disabilities have recognised for themselves (People First 1991; Powerhouse 1996a). However, this is not to call for all, or even most, learning disability services to be segregated by gender, not least because this strategy does nothing to protect men from being sexually abused by other men, which is also a significant problem in learning disability services (Brown, Turk and Stein 1995; McCarthy and Thompson 1997). Moreover, in suggesting changes for the future, it is essential to keep an eye on the past – it is only relatively recently that strict gender segregation was in operation as a matter of course in learning disability services. It is potentially very damaging to the public image and self-image of people with learning disabilities to suggest that gender segregation is always appropriate. Also, many people with learning disabilities, including women, want mixed sex services (Namdarkhan 1995).

Nevertheless, for those men who pose a particular risk to women, and for those women who would prefer a women-only environment, the option of single-sex services should be available. If they are not made available, learning disability services are, in effect, implementing policies which compel women to live with, often, quite large numbers of men. This can lead to a kind of 'siege mentality' developing amongst women with learning disabilities where staff advise them to always lock themselves in their bedrooms (Namdarkhan 1995). It must also be remembered that in certain kinds of services, especially assessment and treatment services and secure services, the term 'mixed services' hides the reality that women are often significantly outnumbered by men – for example, in October 1996 I visited a secure service for people with learning disabilities and found that it housed nineteen men and two women; one woman I worked with (not included in this study) who lived in a RSU was, in fact, the only woman on a ward full of men. Even where the gender imbalance is not at these extreme levels, I believe there are still strong grounds for challenging a policy which obliges vulnerable women to live, work and relax alongside men they have not chosen, are not related to by family or intimate ties and amongst whom there will almost definitely be those with known histories of sexual violence against women.

Changing the law

If there is one area of policy reform that is in urgent need of attention, it is the inadequate response of the legal system as it applies to sexual crimes committed against women (and, indeed, men) with learning disabilities. There is ample evidence that the existing law is failing women with learning disabilities: in this study, despite many sexual crimes being committed against the women, only one of the perpetrators was brought to justice and that was many years ago; in my other research on sexual abuse of people with learning disabilities (McCarthy and Thompson 1997), only 3 out of 59 perpetrators (5%) of sexual abuse against women with learning disabilities were convicted; Turk and Brown indicate that a criminal prosecution or staff disciplinary took place in only 18.5 per cent of cases of sexual abuse against women and men with learning disabilities in their 1992 study and that this figure actually dropped to 14 per cent in their later follow-up study (Brown, Stein and Turk 1995).

It is, of course, the case that where sexual crimes are concerned, the existing legal system fails to give adequate redress to women, regardless of whether they have a disability or not. The many structural imbalances of the current legal system which operate in favour of men accused of rape and other serious sexual crimes have been well documented by Lees (1996). Many of the sexist attitudes held by members of the judiciary, as well as the procedural unfairnesses which Lees highlights, are likely to disadvantage women with learning disabilities even more than other women. For instance, Lees reports that, despite it not being official Home Office policy to do so, police officers 'no-crime' reports of rape if they consider the woman complainant to be unreliable (p.98). This will work to the detriment of women with learning disabilities because it is widely acknowledged that both the police and the Crown Prosecution Service (CPS) tend to view people with learning disabilities as inherently unreliable or 'incompetent' witnesses – a principle Crown prosecutor has admitted as much: 'I won't defend the indefensible; we and the police do back off due to prejudice' (Jackson quoted in Cohen 1994, p.20).

The counsel for the prosecution, who, in lay terms, is perceived to be 'on the woman's side' during rape trials, is, in fact, there to defend the public interest on behalf of the Crown and in no sense can be argued to be playing the same role for the woman as the defence lawyers play for the accused man. In fact, the counsel for the prosecution is not allowed to meet or speak to the woman before the trial and this is, in the view of many people, quite outrageously unfair. Again, although this is detrimental to all women who have been raped, it is likely to particularly disadvantage women with learning disabilities – it is difficult to see how the prosecuting counsel can put anything useful across to a jury about a learning disabled woman's character, capabilities and limitations without ever having met her.

Lees argues that the long delay in rape trials coming to court puts pressure on women in various ways. This is undoubtedly so and, once again, is likely to be especially disadvantageous to women with learning disabilities, who may well have trouble remembering precise details about events in the more distant past and who often have particular trouble being accurate about times and dates (Sone 1995). In addition, it seems likely that women with learning disabilities, like 'psychiatric patients' (Lees 1996, p.111) – indeed, many women with learning disabilities are both – would come into a special category of persons about whom judges have the discretion to give special caution regarding the danger of convicting without uncorroborated evidence, thus stacking the dice even further against them in court.

Although not specifically in relation to sexual crimes, the government has produced a report on the treatment of vulnerable witnesses (Home Office 1998) which contains several recommendations for measures designed to increase the chances of achieving justice for adults with learning disabilities, as well as others who are vulnerable for different reasons. The measures include action which could be taken during police investigations, before and during trials. At the time of writing, this document was under consultation and it remains to be seen whether the recommendations are acted upon and, indeed, whether they prove to be effective.

As well as changes to the existing laws and legal processes, two other legal changes have been suggested as the way to improve matters for people with learning disabilities. The first of these is to rely less on the criminal law and make better use of the civil law. Carson (1994) has argued this case strongly, suggesting that where the CPS decides against bringing a criminal prosecution, a claim for compensation for trespass against the person could be brought in a civil court. He also suggests the possibility of suing learning disability services for failing to protect their clients against sexual abuse or for failing to equip clients with the necessary assertiveness skills so that they would have had a better chance of protecting themselves.

It seems a sensible recommendation to look towards the civil courts, not least because the burden of proof is a lesser one – cases are decided on the 'balance of probabilities' as opposed to 'beyond all reasonable doubt' in the criminal court. However, Carson's suggestions are in themselves problematic for a number of reasons. First, they involve an acceptance that the criminal justice system fails people with learning disabilities and this means that perpetrators of crimes against them will effectively get off with, at most, a fine. Second, they are problematic because although the idea of suing learning disability services is attractive in some ways, it overlooks the important question of who precisely is going to sue. Many people with learning disabilities would be unable to do so themselves; some may have families willing to sue but many families would be reluctant due to fears of losing essential support services and fears of possible unpleasant re-percussions for the service user; independent advocates could well play a role here, although relatively few people with learning disabilities have them. Third, suing a service for having failed to equip people with learning disabilities with assertiveness skills is fraught with problems. Learning disability services would probably defend themselves by saying that they did teach assertiveness skills and that it was, therefore, a deficiency in the individual that made them unwilling or unable to put their teaching into practice. Unseemly wrangles in court about whose fault it was and victim-blaming seem inevitable.

The second fundamental change would be to create a new law which specifically recognises the inherent vulnerability of adults with learning disabilities. To some extent this already exists in the Section 7 of the Sexual Offences Act 1956, which states that a woman with a severe mental impairment is not capable of giving consent to sexual intercourse. But proposals have been made for the creation of a new offence of exploiting a person with a mental disorder (Carson 1994, p.134). Other countries have already gone down this road. For example, in India proposals were made so that the sexual assault of a 'woman who is suffering from a mental or physical disability' should count as an aggravated sexual assault (Khanna and Kapur 1996, p.40); in New South Wales, Australia, the sexual assault of a person with a 'serious physical disability' or a 'serious mental disability' (Rosser 1990, p.34) already counts as an aggravating circumstance for which an extra six years imprisonment can be given. Legally acknowledging the very real vulnerability of many adults with learning disabilities may go some way towards changing public opinion, which is either very ignorant about the lives of people with learning disabilities or seems to overlook their existence altogether. For instance, in a recent special series of articles on child sexual abuse a newspaper journalist wrote the stark sentence 'Children are conned by their abusers in a way that *no adult would be*' (Davies 1998, my emphasis). He went on to give examples of children being bribed by men with tickets to football matches, fast food and sweets. The reality is that many adults with learning disabilities are 'conned' in exactly the same way – adult women with learning disabilities with whom I have worked have been bribed into sex with complete strangers for a bag of sweets or 50p or a ride in a car. This is reported elsewhere in the literature (McCarthy 1993) and men who offer such small incentives are, if prosecuted, often acquitted of any crime. In this country and abroad judges have directed juries to conclude that effectively a fair exchange has taken place (McSherry 1998).

Although such legal changes are welcomed by many, they are also problematic for various reasons. First, legally defining a 'serious' disability will be as difficult with the new laws as it is with existing ones. As Rosser (1990) points out, in practice this will mean that as well as the trauma of having to give evidence about sexual assault, a woman will also have to suffer the indignity of having lawyers argue in court about how able/disabled she is. Second, if women are legally defined as having serious intellectual disabilities, not only might this impact negatively on the way others perceive their ability to make decisions about their lives in a broader context, but it will also suggest to the court that they are unreliable witnesses, thus reducing the chances of securing a conviction, the precise opposite of what is intended. Third, the wider implications of such legislation have been largely overlooked – that is, what it will do to the public image and self-image of people with learning disabilities to be considered so different from other adults that it is automatically considered worse to sexually assault a person with, rather than without, a disability, which is, after all, what making it an aggravating circumstance implies. More debate is needed on these subjects, including hearing what people with learning disabilities think about them.

Provision of sexuality support to people with learning disabilities

The final recommendation for policy change relates to the provision of sexuality support to people who use learning disability services. The aim of all sexuality policies and guidelines should always be to support people with learning disabilities in their sexual lives, not to dissuade them from having sex. The only justification for dissuading people from having sex is if the risks they pose to themselves or others are very serious and cannot be reduced by any other means. Generally speaking, however, this is not the case. In confirming the view that when people are in difficulties they generally need help and support, not removing from the situation, Brown (1983) has stated: 'we do not deal with the issue of bad manners by persuading people not to eat' (p.134). Although I agree with her, I think this is a wrong analogy because people will die if they do not eat but not if they do not have sex (although, judging by some of the writings on this in the 1970s (see p.58), one would think this was the case!). Unlike eating, sex is not a life or death matter, it is a quality of life issue. It is, therefore, entirely appropriate that learning disability services should have policies which address the provision of sexuality support.

In this study a number of the women made it clear that staff were not readily available to them to discuss sexual matters. As many people with learning disabilities have a wide variety of needs in relation to sexual matters (McCarthy 1996b), every learning disability day and residential service should seek to ensure that at least some staff are ready, willing and able to take on this role. This needs to be a policy as well as a practice issue because it has resource implications – for example, for staff training, the purchase of educational materials and, very importantly, staff time. As well as the provision of support for all on an informal basis, all people with learning disabilities should have access to formal sex education as a matter of right. This is not to say that it should be compulsory because there will inevitably be some people who are uninterested and unwilling to attend. However, only five of the seventeen women in this study said that they had received any formal sex education (not including that which they received from me) – this despite the fact that these were all sexually active women who were both motivated and able to discuss the issues.

Sexuality policies should ensure that *proactive* support is given to people with learning disabilities. This means that issues related to sexuality, sexual abuse and sexual health should be routinely discussed as part of Individual Programme Plans (IPPs) or Individual Care Plans (ICPs) and reviewed at regular intervals (Cambridge and McCarthy 1997). Of course, this would need to be done sensitively and in ways which balance the individual's rights to privacy and confidentiality with their need for support (Thompson and Brown 1998). However, making sexuality issues a 'legitimate' part of a service's response to all service users moves away from the reluctant stance still prevalent in many services where sexuality is still only grudgingly addressed for particular individuals who are then, often, viewed as especially troubled or troublesome.

There is conflicting evidence as to whether and how far sex education can protect people from abuse – Hard and Plumb (1986) claim that it did seem to serve a protective function for the people in their study whilst Stromsness (1993) claimed that 'sex education appeared not to prevent abuse, but instead appeared to increase the reporting of sexual abuse' (p.139). In this study formal sex education did not seem to have served a protective function for the five women who received it as they were all subsequently sexually abused. However, it is important to remember the *content* as well as the *existence* of sex education – merely being taught about menstruation and reproduction, as most of these women were, is not likely to protect anyone from sexual abuse.

Despite doubts about the efficacy of sex education (see p.252–253 for recommendations on further research needed in this area), it is accepted that without raising the awareness of individuals 'they may respond indiscriminately to what is asked of them, be unaware of appropriate behaviour, possess poor judgement in sizing up the motivations of others or act impulsively' (Kiehlbauch Cruz, Price-Williams and Andron 1988, p.414). Hingsburger's book *Just Say Know!* (1995), is built around the central theme of the importance of sex education for people with learning disabilities as a protective strategy. Although sex education which teaches self-protection strategies is of limited effectiveness (because it is an individualised approach to what is essentially a social problem), it is still, nevertheless, important that people with learning disabilities have access to it. It is also important that service providers realise its limitations and be prepared to try to minimise risks in other, more systemic ways (McCarthy and Thompson 1996).

Although this research, and, indeed, the whole body of my work in this field, is concerned with the sexuality of adults with learning disabilities, I am not unaware of the needs of children with learning disabilities in this area. Sex education, in its broadest sense, needs to begin at an early age. Children with learning disabilities, like other children, need structured teaching and informal support to learn that their bodies belong to them and that they have the right not to be abused. They also need to learn that their bodies can be sources of pleasure and about appropriate social and sexual behaviour. Whilst parents clearly have an important role here, so do schools. There are some excellent examples of special schools and innovative projects which teach personal safety and sexuality issues to pupils with varying degrees of learning disabilities (Craft *et al.* 1996; Scott *et al.* 1994; Stewart 1993). Equipping children and young people with the knowledge and skills that will be useful to them throughout their adult lives should be seen as a priority.

Practice recommendations

Delivery of sex education and broader sexuality support to women with learning disabilities

At the end of Chapter One I argued that it was only a feminist perspective which allowed a proper understanding of the gendered nature of power relations between men and women with learning disabilities. Thus, in making any recommendations about the delivery of sex education, an understanding of power issues is crucial. Thomson (1994) comes to the same conclusion with regard to sex education of young people at school: 'For sex education to be meaningful it needs to address and develop moral autonomy and to do this it needs to address power and inter-connecting relationships of power' (p.55).

Central to understanding gender power relations is the awareness that heterosexual women and men (whether they have learning disabilities or not) very often lead quite different sexual lives (Crawford *et al.* 1994; Holland *et al.* 1993; McCarthy 1994). Therefore, it is unlikely that exactly the same sex education, advice and support will be useful to both men and women.

The different motivations for women and men with learning disabilities to engage in sexual activity with each other needs to be better understood, both by people with learning disabilities themselves and those who support them. In another recent piece of research on the sexuality of people with learning disabilities I found that, whilst 49 per cent of women (n=65) had had sex with a man or men without really wanting or enjoying it in its own right (i.e. they were induced, coerced or felt it necessary to develop or maintain a relationship), only 1 per cent of men (n=120) had had sex with a woman without really wanting to (McCarthy 1996b). This fits very much into the gendered stereotypes of women wanting boyfriends and men wanting sex (Holland *et al.* 1990). Whilst these are uncomfortable stereotypes (and, of course, not true for all women and men), they, nevertheless, still seem to apply to many people. As long as this is still the case, it indicates that great emphasis needs to be placed on self-esteem and assertiveness work for women with learning disabilities. This is not just in relation to sexual matters but more generally. Indeed, it is unrealistic to expect women (with or without learning disabilities) to become sexually assertive with men before they are more generally assertive (Dickson 1985). The only hope for women to be able to get and keep what they want in a relationship and not constantly be giving men what men want is if they can become sufficiently assertive to negotiate from a position of strength. Obviously, in the longer term, one can only hope that these polarised positions of many men and women would converge. Learning disability services could help women in this respect by assisting the women to lead fuller, more independent lives with better social networks and with a variety of interesting and stimulating activities. As long as the most, and, sometimes, the only, valued thing in a woman's life is her relationship with a man, this leaves her emotionally dependent and vulnerable.

One of the most stark and depressing conclusions from this research and my broader work with women with learning disabilities is the lack of sexual pleasure they get from much, and, in some cases, all, of their sexual activity with men. This was also found by Andron and Ventura (1987), Millard (1994), and by Holland *et al.* (1990) and Thompson (1990) in their research on non-disabled young women in Britain and the USA. However, the widespread lack of sexual pleasure for women is not well understood within learning disability services. Simplistic assumptions get made that if a woman is having a lot of sex, she must be enjoying it, otherwise she would not do it. But the fact remains that there is not necessarily any direct correlation between the amount of sex and/or sexual partners and the amount of sexual pleasure a woman experiences (Russell 1995).

However, very few women with learning disabilities have complained about not experiencing sexual pleasure, in this study or at other times, and it could, therefore, be argued that it is non-disabled people involved in sex education, myself included, who are imposing our priorities on them. To some extent this is true, but it is equally true of many other aspects of life for people with learning disabilities – because of low expectations and low self-esteem, very often people do not complain, nor, indeed, realise that life could be better.

It therefore seems that there is a very strong case for recommending that all sex education work with women with learning disabilities should place a significant emphasis on women's sexual pleasure. In practical terms this would mean emphasising the sexual pleasure that women could get from masturbation and informing women that this could help them learn what kind of sexual stimulation they might welcome from their sexual partners. That an emphasis on education about the acceptability (and, indeed, widespread prevalence) of non-penetrative activities during heterosexual sex is needed was clearly shown by the women in this study. For example, in answer to a question about whether they engaged in mutual masturbation with men, a number of women answered along the lines of:

> This is not proper sex, because men are getting you to do wrong, naughty things before they get down to the basics. (MC)

> I wouldn't like doing it, I've been brought up different. (MH)

The potential for, and pleasures in, lesbian partnerships and sexual activity should also have a more prominent place in sex education work with women. Whilst nobody should be directed towards any one form of sexual experience, including heterosexuality, it is appropriate to open up options for people. Sex between men with learning disabilities is much more common than sex between women and I have explained why I think this is (see p.204). I have justified elsewhere why I think women with learning disabilities might benefit from learning more about the possibilities of relationships with other women:

> Given the unsatisfactory nature of much of the heterosexual activity for many women with learning disabilities, it is of concern that it seems, for whatever reasons, to be less possible for them to engage in same sex activity and relationships than it is for their male peers. Relationships with other women might offer them the pleasure and satisfaction that the women often reported were absent in their relationships with men.

However the downside would be that the women would be faced with the stresses related to homophobia that many men with learning disabilities currently face. (McCarthy 1996b, p.275)

Sex education needs to emphasise a more active, less passive and accepting role for women with learning disabilities. This may mean, for some women, taking the initiative and at least some of the control. But accepting that this is likely to be very difficult for many women who have absorbed the more traditional gendered stereotypes about sexual roles, at a more basic level it could also mean taking decisions, standing up for oneself and trying to resist pressure.

In Thompson's (1990) research with non-disabled young women, she found that those who experienced sex negatively 'didn't look ahead to sex. They didn't prepare. They didn't explore. Often they didn't even agree to sex. They gave in, they gave up, they gave out' (p.351). She also found that those who experienced sex positively had previous and ongoing experience of masturbation and had experienced orgasm through that. They also had more non-penetrative sex than the others. They also had mothers and other older women around them who talked positively about enjoying sex. As Thompson says, 'They had learnt a lesson that ...is crucial: that women can be the subjects of their own desire' (p.354). The positive role models and messages that this group of young women had are very important and something that sex education could try to emulate. It is essential to make it socially acceptable for women to talk positively about enjoying their sexual activity. Without that, it will remain very difficult for women to experience and understand their sexual experiences positively. This has been long understood – as Wolf (1997) shows in her analysis of Margaret Mead's anthropological work from the 1940s, three cultural factors are important if women are to be able to experience their sexuality positively. These are:

1. She must live in a culture that recognises female desire as being of value.

2. Her culture must allow her to understand the mechanics of her sexual anatomy.

3. Her culture must teach the various skills that can make women experience orgasm. (Wolf 1997, p.9)

However, unlike for men, there is no positive discourse for women which permits them to describe sexual experiences (including masturbation) which they really wanted at the time, thoroughly enjoyed and are looking forward to repeating (Thomson 1996). Indeed, if women, especially girls and young women, do express positive views about sex, they risk being labelled as a 'slag' or 'slut' and ruining their reputations (Lees 1993, 1997). In formal contexts, such as schools (Fine 1988), and for adults with learning disabilities (Millard 1994), there is a 'missing discourse' of female sexual desire (Fine 1988). However, many writers have suggested that the influence of feminism(s) can help to create discourses which allow for women's power and desire to be positively described and experienced (see Gavey 1992; Segal 1994; Plummer 1995).

Thompson (1990) suggests that in order to bring the women who experienced sex negatively closer to those who had positive experiences, what we have traditionally thought of as 'sex education' needs to be reframed as 'erotic education' (p.357). Although the phrase 'erotic education' is unfamiliar and sounds a little odd, the content of what Thompson proposes for young women is very similar to that which I suggest above for women with learning disabilities.

The fundamental change I am recommending to the way women with learning disabilities are supported in their sexual lives focuses on the women's empowerment. This kind of empowerment is most likely to be achieved by helping women with learning disabilities to engage in a process of critical reflection about their sexual lives. This is something I have been attempting to do, with the women in this study and others, over the past eight years. I say that I have been attempting to do it because, in reality, it is extremely difficult to do, not least because some women do not want to do it (see, for example, my discussion with DY on p.180). Reflecting on one's past behaviour or experiences can be painful and threatening to one's sense of self. Nevertheless, if women have the courage and support to do it, it can be beneficial. The kind of critical reflection I am referring to is what Holland *et al.* (1991b) call 'intellectual empowerment'. They suggest, as I do, that critically reflecting on past sexual experiences, especially where these were pressured or otherwise negative experiences, can lead women to desire a different and more positive experience in future sexual encounters.

However, Holland *et al.* (1991b) emphasise that empowerment at the intellectual level – that is, women deciding that they want things to be different 'is insufficient to ensure that women can act effectively on their positive conceptions' (p.23). Sheer acts of personal will are not enough. They suggest that women need also 'to be *empowered at an experiential level*' (p.19, original emphasis). This means women being able to put their ideas into practice and achieve a shift in male dominance. In other words, for women to be able to change their feelings, beliefs and experiences of sex, men also need to change. This is because, with the best will in the world, 'feminism cannot direct women into secure or happy relationships with reconstructed men. Such relationships require men to reflect critically on their masculinity' (Ramazanoglu 1992, p.446). This is extremely important as, otherwise, the situation may well develop for some women with learning disabilities as it has for other women – that is, becoming empowered and resolving not to put up with poor treatment from men may well lead to not finding or sustaining relationships with male partners at all. This in itself can then lead to a loss of self-esteem. As Ramazanoglu has memorably put it 'Political correctness is no comfort on a lonely Saturday night' (p.445).

Delivery of sex education and broader sexuality support to men with learning disabilities

In terms of changing things for the better for women with learning disabili-ties, I am in absolutely no doubt that efforts must be put into helping men change their sexual behaviour. There are some areas where it would be useful to give explicit and specific advice to men with learning disabilities. For example, men need to be told not to concentrate only on penetrative sex; that they should avoid anal penetration and penis-oral contact unless they get a clear signal from women that they want this (the justification for this is that these are the two sexual activities disliked most by the vast majority of women with learning disabilities I have spoken to); men need to be made aware of the need for, and ways to ensure, some natural or artificial lubrica-tion before penetration (using lubricated condoms could help here and, in any event, use of condoms needs to be encouraged for sexual health reasons); men need to be told what and where the clitoris is and what the purpose is of them stimulating it (i.e. they need to be explicitly introduced to the idea of the giving sexual pleasure to a woman – as Gerrard (1998) has recently writ-ten in relation to 'man's search for the clitoris...things aren't just discovered. They have to be needed as well' (p.3)); men with learning disabilities also need to be educated into not ceasing all sexual activity the moment they have sexually satisfied themselves through orgasm; that they should not offer financial or other bribes or inducements to get women to engage in sex with them; and that they should never pressure or force a woman (or, indeed, another man) to have sex.

In addition to that detailed level of advice, men with learning disabilities need more general education about relating sexually to women – that is, understanding the importance of mutuality, respect and not always putting their own needs first. Put more starkly, men with learning disabilities, like other men, need to start choosing *not* to take what they want sexually or what they perceive themselves to need or be entitled to. They need to learn that, however easy it might be to avail themselves of it, they do not have the *right* of sexual access to anybody. As Jensen (1996) states: 'The simple truth is that in this culture men have to make a conscious decision not to rape, because rape is so readily available to us and so rarely results in sanctions of any kind' (p.96). Looked at in this way, it is clear that men need to learn to negotiate just as much as women do.

Those men with learning disabilities who continue to overstep the boundaries of acceptable sexual behaviour need to be given a clear message that this will not be tolerated. Both punishment and support/treatment for the offending behaviour seem appropriate here (Thompson and Brown 1998). However, in reality, legal sanctions against men with learning disabilities who sexually offend against women with learning disabilities are rarely applied. Thompson (1997) has shown that men with learning disabilities are only legally punished when they sexually offend against children or non-disabled women (e.g. members of the public) and not when the victims are other people (men or women) with learning disabilities. This was despite the fact that the sexual offences committed against people with learning disabilities were generally more serious offences than those against the other groups.

Not punishing men with learning disabilities for sexual offences against other people with learning disabilities gives a message that it is acceptable. I have acknowledged earlier that the law is very weak at dealing with sexual offences and that there is evidence to suggest that suspects and defendants with learning disabilities are at a disadvantage at various stages of the criminal justice system. Therefore, it is also appropriate and necessary for learning disability services themselves to apply sanctions against men who sexually offend (Thompson and Brown 1998), although this is ethically, and sometimes practically, very difficult. However, this is not a view shared by everyone – for example, in a book which is excellent in its analysis of the seriousness of crimes committed against people with learning disabilities and in its argument to bring the perpetrators to justice, Williams (1995) makes an exception where the perpetrators of crimes have learning disabilities and suggests that police could be asked to have informal discussions, give warnings or cautions. No cogent argument is made as to the justification for this. In addition, he states that there is no place for services to take any action of their own: 'if an offence cannot be proven, no action can be taken against an alleged perpetrator' (p.24). This entirely overlooks the structural injustices of the legal system which mean that it is relatively rare for a sexual offence to be proven (Lees 1996) and leaves learning disability services to struggle on trying to manage both an alleged perpetrator and victim in the same service. My own view is that despite the inherent weaknesses of the criminal justice system and despite the dangers of men with learning disabilities potentially being disadvantaged in comparison to other suspects and defendants, it is wrong to avoid applying the law to them when they sexually offend against women with learning disabilities (see also Thompson and Brown 1998); this seems defeatist and will ultimately work against the interests of women.

Not applying sanctions, legal or otherwise, when men with learning disabilities sexually abuse others means that, effectively, male dominated institutions (health authorities, social service departments, police, courts) are condoning their behaviour. However, I realise that challenging male service users about their sexual behaviour is not an easy thing to do. Within learning disability services, individuals who attempt such challenges are accused by others of being too authoritarian, oppressive and wanting to take away rights to sexual expression. However, experienced practitioners and researchers maintain:

> …one factor we noted which allowed men with learning disabilities to fail to appreciate the seriousness of their behaviour was that responses and sanctions have been too infrequently and inconsistently applied to them. Men might have learned to stop what they were doing if the responses had been immediate, clear and firm (Thompson and Brown 1998, p.108).

In suggesting that efforts need to be made to get men with learning disabilities to change their sexual attitudes and behaviour towards women, I am very aware that it is a limited approach because women with learning disabilities also have sex with men who do not have any kind of disability. It is rare that learning disability services have any significant contact with these men and, even if they did, it is hard to imagine that they would welcome sex education or advice from these services. My only attempt at doing this work myself (a woman with mild learning disabilities requested that I talk to her boyfriend who was very much more intellectually able than her and he agreed because they had a sexual problem he wanted to resolve) was not a great success – in fact, it was unpleasant for me and frustrating for both the man and myself. He was solely concerned with what he perceived as his girlfriend's problem – that is, her not wanting or being able to experience vaginal penetration to his satisfaction. I, not surprisingly, wanted to take a rather broader view of what was and was not happening between them sexually and otherwise. There was no common ground between us – he left, patently insulted that I had implied it was at least as much his problem as hers, telling me my advice was rubbish, and I was left feeling concerned at his attitude to, and treatment of, women and what this would mean for any woman he became sexually involved with.

However, the fact that not all the potential sexual partners of women with learning disabilities can be reached (in all senses of the word) should not prevent services from doing what they can with those with whom it is possible.

Who should deliver sex education to people with learning disabilities?

Elsewhere (McCarthy and Thompson 1992; McCarthy 1994), I have suggested that the more formal forms of sex education, such as one-to-one work or group sessions, are best done on a single-sex basis. I would re-emphasise this in the recommendations here. A same-gender approach when discussing matters of a highly personal and intimate nature is a logical extension of the widely accepted (although by no means universally implemented) practice of providing a member of staff of the same sex for assistance with personal care tasks – for example, washing, dressing, help with bodily functions such as going to the toilet and, for women, with periods. A same-gender approach to discussing sexual matters also offers a greater chance to the person with learning disabilities to identify with the person trying to advise and support them. In addition, it offers, where appropriate, the opportunity to look at some shared life experiences, as this study has illustrated.

From a feminist point of view, this approach has the added advantage of giving male workers the responsibility for addressing men's sexuality and sexual abuse. However, this approach has practical shortcomings because male workers are under-represented in learning disability services and are further under-represented amongst those who take an active interest in sexuality issues (McCarthy and Thompson 1996; Malhotra and Mellan 1996). Nevertheless, my recommendation would be that planners and managers of learning disability services adopt a strategy whereby they actively encourage and support male workers rather than passively accepting that women staff are 'naturally' going to be more interested and skilled at this work.

The involvement of people with learning disabilities themselves in the delivery of peer sex education is an important area which goes largely undiscussed in the literature or field more broadly (see Barber and Redfern 1997 for an exception). It is even more unusual to find any critique of this aspect of sex education (see McCarthy and Thompson 1995 for an exception). People with learning disabilities educating and supporting their peers on sexual issues has the potential to be a powerful tool for change – members of other disadvantaged groups have chosen to work with others who share at least some of their characteristics and life experiences and there is no reason to think that some people with learning disabilities would not also benefit from being able to do the same. Also, non-disabled people, most importantly professionals, benefit from learning from people with learning disabilities. There are some excellent examples of people with learning disabilities acting as educators, trainers and advocates (see, for example, Powerhouse 1996; *Colour Me Loud* video 1994).

However, whilst there may be advantages in a peer education approach, it should also be acknowledged that if people with learning disabilities are to become more involved in the delivery of sex education, they (like others) will need training, support and supervision. Just because having sex is an ordinary life experience does not mean that anybody can be a sex educator. Helping people understand their own and other people's sexuality and, where appropriate, make changes in their sexual behaviour is a complex and skilled task and if it is to be done properly it calls for those involved to have the following attributes:

- good listening and communication skills
- to be knowledgeable about a wide variety of sexual practices and lifestyles
- to have an open mind and be able to empathise with the situations and behaviours of others
- to be able to assimilate complex information and, in turn, be flexible in how information and advice is given out

- to be able to develop an understanding about why people behave in ways that are harmful to themselves and others

- to be able to help people develop strategies to overcome their difficulties

- to understand the effect of a person's history and environment on their current and future sexual behaviour

- to be patient and prepared to persevere despite little or no evidence of change over time

- to be able to make selective use of available sex education materials

- to know one's own limits and when to refer people elsewhere

- to be able to involve key people from a person's network where such support is necessary but, at the same time, maintain appropriate boundaries of confidentiality

- to act as advocates for better support services for individuals and groups.

If people with learning disabilities have most or all of the above skills, this, in combination with the unique insights they can bring from their shared experience of having an intellectual impairment, would undoubtedly make them excellent sex educators. But it is important not to lose sight of the skills involved in the task. After all, we do not hear much debate about peer psychology or peer dentistry as it is recognised that the skills involved effectively rule out those with a learning disability (Thompson, personal communication). However, if it is true that professionals can do certain things which people with learning disabilities generally cannot, it is also true the other way around. People who themselves have learning disabilities are, by virtue of living, working, socialising in the same services or geographical area, able to offer continuity and longer term support than many professionals who may come and go. They are also able to validate one another's experiences and are often better able than professionals to understand the circumstances of everyday life and, therefore, the priorities of their peers. A poignant example of this was my own experience of being involved in the organisation of the first ever national conference for women with learning disabilities (see Walmsley 1993). The predominantly non-disabled organisers had taken great care to ensure a wide range of workshops to cover sexual abuse, sexual health, women's health issues, a workshop for lesbians and one for Black women, etc. In the event, when women with learning disabilities came to make their choice about workshops, the most popular choice *by far* was a workshop on 'Making Friends'.

Rather than contemplating whether peer educators can offer sex education on the same terms as professionals (with few of the advantages and resources which professionals have at their disposal), it seems more helpful to make clearer distinctions about the roles and purpose of peer and professional involvement. Peer support is not the same as professional sex education but they can complement each other. However, where people with learning disabilities do get involved in actually delivering sex education to their peers, as opposed to providing more informal support, they should be subject to the same scrutiny and evaluation as others. If people with learning disabilities are effectively providing a service to others, for which they may well receive a fee, there are certain minimum standards of 'professional' behaviour which need to be maintained. This does not always happen and, because of fears about being seen to be 'politically incorrect', others, including myself, do not complain in the same way as they would if it were a non-disabled person behaving in that way. One example which I found personally difficult to deal with involved a man with learning disabilities who co-facilitated a conference workshop on sexuality issues. Much of the content of the workshop was about respect for individuals and maintaining appropriate boundaries. Straight after the workshop he approached me in a very inappropriate way, saying 'I like you' and rubbing his head on my upper arm and pushing my hand down towards his lap (he was sitting in a wheelchair). Another example involved a woman with learning disabilities, who was co-facilitating a workshop on safer sex education for other people with learning disabilities, who made several overtly homophobic statements. In my view, neither of these examples meet acceptable standards of behaviour for sex educators. Whilst it is true, in theory, that they could just as easily have been carried out by non-disabled sex educators, in practice, I have not seen similar behaviour from professionals, despite long experience in this field. It is my view that people with learning disabilities have a right to sexuality support from others (whether they have a learning disability or not) who have an understanding of, and a commitment to challenge, various forms of sexual inequality and who attempt to apply these principles to their own practice.

Although it feels very difficult to criticise the work of people with learning disabilities (so difficult, in fact, that it is practically never done by professionals in public, although it is in private), there are occasions when I feel criticism is justified. For example, the book *Women First: A Book by Women with Learning Difficulties* about the issues for women with learning difficulties (People First, undated but publicly launched at the end of 1996) has a section on sexuality. The clitoris is missing from the diagram of women's 'sexual/ sensitive parts' (p.17) and sex itself is described in the following way:

> Sex is something that we can choose to have with our boyfriends or girlfriends. We all have the right to choose if we want to do this or not. Sex can mean lots of things from kissing and cuddling to actual sexual intercourse. Sexual intercourse is when a man puts his penis into the woman's vagina. The man gets very excited and comes in the woman's vagina. When this happens the man's sperm could make the woman have a baby. (p.18)

Although it is encouraging that the women have included the possibility of lesbian sex and non-penetrative sexual activities, it is very disappointing that they completely omit any reference to women's sexual excitement and orgasm. In addition, the only pictures of sexual activity in the book show vaginal intercourse with the man on top of the woman. It is difficult to know quite why information about women's sexual pleasure has been omitted – it is hard to believe that the women with learning disabilities involved in producing the book had the knowledge themselves but deliberately chose to withhold it from other women. It seems more likely that either they were too embarrassed to include it or they simply did not know it themselves – that is, they lacked the awareness and skills to be able to look beyond their own range of experiences. In common with some other publications on sexual issues by people with learning disabilities, for example *Everything You Ever Wanted to Know about Safer Sex…But Nobody Bothered to Tell You* (People First undated), individuals have not put their names to their work, thus making it harder to enquire as to why something was included or omitted.

Final recommendations and concluding remarks

Like all research, this study has been limited and some areas of investigation have been overlooked. Consequently, a general recommendation is that further research needs to be carried out in the whole area of women's sexuality.

There are six specific recommendations for further research: first, the experiences of Black women with learning disabilities are missing from this study, for the reasons outlined on p.121. Therefore, the sexual lives and sexual abuse of Black women with learning disabilities should be investigated in their own right and by way of comparison with the experiences of white women which are reported in this study and elsewhere in the literature.

Second, the experiences of women with learning disabilities who relate sexually to other women are also missing from this study. Although it would be difficult to find a big enough sample group to study, it should not be impossible and it is important so that services know how to support lesbians with learning disabilities.

Third, the consented sexual experiences of women with learning disabilities who have not also been sexually abused are largely missing from this study and, indeed, most others. Once again, it would be difficult to find a big enough sample group to study but, nevertheless it is important to do so because only in this way will it be possible to investigate whether, and how, women with learning disabilities who have not been abused experience their sexual lives more positively.

Fourth, this study has focused very much on what women with learning disabilities do sexually and what they think and feel about that. It has, therefore, only marginally addressed the broader, but, nevertheless, very important, issues related to women's sexuality – for example, issues around fertility and reproduction. Therefore, it is a recommendation that these become research topics in their own right.

Fifth, it is recommended that some longitudinal research takes place with women (and men) with learning disabilities to evaluate what impact, if any, sex education and sexuality support actually has on their lives in the longer term. Currently, this is under-researched and consequently not well understood.

Finally, it is recommended that the influence of gender upon the lives of girls and boys, women and men with learning disabilities becomes a subject of research in much broader areas than sexuality. This is becoming more frequent now than it once was. However, it is interesting to note that, aside from work which has sexuality as its underlying topic of investigation, other work about *gender* is, in fact, almost exclusively about *women* (e.g. Noonan Walsh 1988; Williams 1992; Burns 1993; Brown 1996. See Hazlehurst 1993 and Townsley 1995 for rare examples of exploring gender issues with men with learning disabilities). Apart from sexuality issues, the only other area of work where gender issues are beginning to be explored is the challenging behaviour of people with learning disabilities (e.g. Clements,

Clare and Ezelle 1995). The importance of understanding the impact of gender upon the totality of a person with learning disabilities' life experience is emphasised by Clements, Clare and Ezelle when they state 'there is a high cost to be paid if a person is perceived as gender free in a gendered world' (p.426).

At the outset of this research it was my intention to apply some of the principles and practices of qualitative and feminist research methodologies to the investigation of the sexual experiences of women with learning disabilities. I set out to understand in some depth what women with learning disabilities did sexually (and what was done to them) and what the women thought and felt about these experiences. My findings in this study have indicated that the sexual side of adult life was not generally positive, pleasurable or life-enhancing for most the seventeen women represented here. The findings of this study are in line with my own broader experience in this area and what little detailed information there is in the literature about the sexual experiences of women with learning disabilities. This suggests that the recommendations which I have formulated would benefit many women with learning disabilities – both those who are still in, or who may enter, hospitals and those who are now living, or have always lived, in community settings.

Summary of recommendations

Policy recommendations

1. The continuation of the hospital closure programme.

2. Policies to reduce risks of sexual abuse to women in learning disability services; prevent admissions of men with little or no learning disability who have histories of sexual offences; where hospital services do still exist, move regional secure units off-site; provide some women-only residential provision.

3. Every learning disability service to implement a policy which stipulates that formal and informal sexuality support will be provided to the people who use the service.

CHANGES TO THE LAW

1. Remove current structural inequalities that exist between the women who bring charges and the men who defend themselves against them.

2. Bring cases of rape and sexual assault to trial quicker.

3. Increase use of civil law, where appropriate.

4. Give consideration to the creation of a new law which specifically recognises the vulnerability of adults with learning disabilities.

Practice recommendations

1. All sex education and broader sexuality support should be informed by an understanding of gender power relations and the different expectations and constraints which operate for women and men with learning disabilities.

2. All sex education to emphasise women's sexual pleasure.

3. All sex education and assertiveness work with women with learning disabilities needs to take on board the complexities of intellectual and experiential empowerment.

4. All sexuality support in learning disability services should prioritise working with men to the same extent as with women, although recognising that the content will be different in a number of ways.

5. All learning disability services need to develop strategies to prevent and manage the sexual abuse which is perpetrated by men who use the services.

6. A single-sex approach to sex education should be encouraged, except where women with learning disabilities actively want to discuss these issues with men.

7. The provision of training and support in anti-discriminatory practice for those people with learning disabilities who are engaging in peer sex education.

Recommendations for further research

1. To understand the sexual experiences of Black and other ethnic minority women with learning disabilities.

2. To understand the sexual experiences of women with learning disabilities who relate, or wish to relate, sexually to other women.

3. To understand the sexual experiences of women with learning disabilities who have not been sexually abused.

4. To understand what women with learning disabilities think and feel about issues related to their fertility and reproductive rights.

5. Longitudinal research to understand the impact of sex education on the lives of people with learning disabilities.

6. To understand the impact of gender more broadly upon the non-sexual lives of girls and boys, women and men with learning disabilities.

Interview Questions

[NB. The questions would not necessarily have been put to interviewees in the way they are worded here, nor in this exact order.]

Sexual activity

1. Do you like having sex?

2. What do/don't you like about it?

3. Who do you have sex with? If, men, boyfriend, other known men, any man who asks, including men without learning difficulties?

4. Do men like having sex with you? How do you know?

5. Do you masturbate?

6. Is this better/worse/same as having sex with a man or just different?

7. Do you know other women or men who do this? What do you think about this?

8. Do you have sex with women?

9. Is it better/worse/same as having sex with a man or just different?

10. Do you know any other women who have sex with women? On TV? What do you think about this?

11. Do you ever think/dream/fantasise about sex?

12. If you could never have sex again, would you miss it?

13. Do you ever talk to anybody about sex?

14. Do you know what/where your clitoris is? What do you call it?

15. Do you have orgasms? What do you call them? Are the orgasms from masturbation? Sex with men? Sex with women?

16. Does the man have orgasms? How? How do you know?

17. Does sex ever/regularly hurt? Is it supposed to hurt? What do you do when it hurts?

18. What do you usually do when you have sex with a man? Describe activities:

   • vaginal penetration, which position?

   • anal penetration?

   • kissing?

   • touching/masturbating?

   • oral sex (both ways)?

19. If you have penetrative sex (vaginal or anal), is there any lubrication? Natural – how?

   Artificial – what is it?

   None – does it hurt? What do you do if it hurts?

20. Do you have sex during your period?

21. Which sort of sex do you like best? Which do you like least?

   What about oral sex?

22. Which sort of sex do men like best/least?

23. Which sort of sex do you have most/least often?

24. Does any kind of sex scare you?

25. Do men pay you for sex? Do you think men should pay women for sex? What about women paying men?

26. Where do you have sex? Do you think you have enough private places and time for sex? (If no, how would it make a difference if you did have more privacy?)

27. Do you take all/some of your clothes off? Does the man?

28. Who decides what sort of sex you have? Who decides where and when you have it? Who decides when it is over? Do you ever want it to go on longer?

29. Do you choose the man? Does he choose you?

30. Would you ever feel able to ask a man for sex? What circumstances?

31. Why do you have sex with men, e.g. love, good feelings, status, approval, money, etc?

32. Who wants sex the most? You or the man?

33. Has anyone ever forced you to have sex when you didn't want to? Do you know if this has ever happened to anyone else?

34. Have you ever made anyone have sex with you when they didn't want to?

35. Have you/would you ever have sex with a person who was a lot more 'handicapped' than you?

36. Who enjoys sex the most? You or the man?

37. Where/how did you learn about sex? School, parents, friends, partners?

Other people's sex

38. Do you know what sort of sex other people (outside the service) have?

39. Do you think staff/families have sex? Is this the same as you or different? How?

    Do you think they masturbate?

40. When other people have sex, do you think women or men enjoy it more? Why?

41. Do you ever see people on TV/films have sex?

42. What happens? Is this the same as yours or different?

43. Who enjoys it more on TV, men or women? How do you know?

Body image/self-esteem/personal hygiene

44. What do you like about your body?

45. What don't you like about your body?

46. If you could change anything about your body, what would it be?

47. Do any parts of your body give you good feelings?

48. Is it important to keep your body clean?

49. Can you keep as clean as you want?

50. Do other people try to make you have 'too many' baths/washes?

Clothes

51. Who chooses your clothes (to buy and daily dressing)?

52. What kind of clothes do you like?

53. Do your clothes make you feel good/bad/neutral?

Sexual health

54. Have you ever had anything wrong with your private parts? Any infections?

55. Why do you think this happened?

56. Did it worry/embarrass you?

57. Did you tell people about it?

58. What kind of contraception do you use? Who chose this? Are you happy with it?

Sexual being/identity

59. Do you think of yourself as a sexual person (feelings, decisions, etc) or does sex just happen to you?

60. When you're having sex, what makes you feel good/bad about yourself?

61. Is sex important to you?

References

Acker, J., Barry, K. and Esseveld, J. (1983) 'Objectivity and truth: Problems in doing feminist research.' *Women's Studies International Forum 6*, 4, 423–435.

Agar, M. (1985) *Speaking of Ethnography*. Beverly Hills: Sage.

Ames, T. (1991) 'Guidelines for providing sexuality-related services to severely and profoundly retarded individuals: The challenge for the nineteen-nineties.' *Sexuality and Disability 9*, 2, 113–122.

Andron, L. (1983) 'Sexuality counselling with developmentally disabled couples.' In M. Craft and A. Craft (eds) *Sex Education and Counselling for Mentally Handicapped People*. Tunbridge Wells: Costello.

Andron, L. and Ventura, J. (1987) 'Sexual dysfunction in couples with learning handicaps.' *Sexuality and Disability 8*, 1, 25–35.

Andron, L. and Tymchuk, A. (1987) 'Parents who are mentally retarded.' In A. Craft (ed) *Mental Handicap and Sexuality: Issues and Perspectives*. Tunbridge Wells: Costello.

ARC/NAPSAC (1993) *It Could Never Happen Here!* Chesterfield and Nottingham: ARC/NAPSAC.

Arscott, K., Dagnon, D. and Kroese, B.S. (1998) 'Consent to psychological research by people with an intellectual disability.' *Journal of Applied Research in Intellectual Disability 11*, 1, 77–83.

Atkinson, D. (1989) 'Research interviews with people with mental handicaps.' In A. Brechin and J. Walmsley (eds) *Making Connections*. London: Hodder and Stoughton.

Atkinson, D. and Williams, F. (1990) *'Know Me As I Am': An Anthology of Prose, Poetry and Art by People with Learning Difficulties*. London: Hodder and Stoughton.

Bank-Mikkelson, N. (1980) 'Denmark.' In R. Flynn and K. Nitsch (eds) *Normalisation, Social Integration and Community Services*. Austin, Texas: Pro-Ed.

Barber, F. and Redfern, P. (1997) 'Safer sex training for peer educators.' In P. Cambridge and H. Brown (eds) *HIV and Learning Disability*. Kidderminster: BILD Publications.

Barker, D. (1983) 'How to curb the fertility of the unfit: The feeble-minded in Edwardian Britain.' *Oxford Journal of Education 9*, 3, 197–211.

Barrett, M. and McIntosh, M. (1982) *The Anti-Social Family*. London: Verso.

Barry, G. (1994) 'How the police can help.' *NAPSAC Bulletin*, September, 5–8.

Bax, M., Smyth, D. and Thomas, A. (1988) 'Health care of physically handicapped young adults.' *British Medical Journal 296*, 23 April, 1153–5.

Baxter, C., Pooner, K., Ward, L. and Nadirshaw, Z. (1990) *Double Discrimination? Services for People with Learning Disabilities from Black and Ethnic Minority Families*. London: Kings Fund.

Baxter, C. (1994) 'Sex education in the multi-racial society.' In A. Craft (ed) *Practice Issues in Sexuality and Learning Disabilities*. London: Routledge.

Bell, A. and Bhate, M. (1992) 'Prevalence of overweight and obesity in Down's Syndrome and other mentally handicapped adults living in the community.' *Journal of Intellectual Disability Research 36*, 4, 359–364.

Bender, M., Aitman, J., Biggs, S. and Haug, U. (1983) 'Initial findings concerning a sexual knowledge questionnaire.' *Mental Handicap 11,* December, 168–169.

Blacker, C. (1950) *Eugenics in Retrospect and Prospect: The Galton Society Lecture 1945.* London: The Eugenics Society and Cassell & Co. Ltd. (2nd Edition).

Bland, L. (1995) *Banishing the Beast: English Feminism and Sexual Morality 1885–1914.* London: Penguin.

Bone, M., Spain, B. and Fox, M. (1972) *Plans and Provision for the Mentally Handicapped.* London: George Allen and Unwin.

Booth, T. and Booth, W. (1992) 'Practice in sexuality.' *Mental Handicap 20,* 2, 64–69.

Booth, T. and Booth, W. (1994) *Parenting Under Pressure: Mothers and Fathers with Learning Difficulties.* Buckingham: Open University Press.

Booth, T. and Booth, W. (1995) 'For better, for worse: Professional practice and parents with learning difficulties.' In T. Philpot and L. Ward (eds) *Values and Visions: Changing Ideas in Services for People with Learning Difficulties.* Oxford: Butterworth-Heinemann.

Brannen, J. and Collard, J. (1982) *Marriages in Trouble: The Process of Seeking Help.* London: Tavistock.

Breakwell, G. (1986) *Coping with Threatened Identities.* London: Methuen.

Brecher, E. (1972) *The Sex Researchers.* London: Panther.

Brewer, J. (1993) 'Sensitivity as a problem in field research: A study of routine policing in Northern Ireland.' In C. Renzetti and R. Lee (eds) *Researching Sensitive Topics.* London: Sage Publications.

Brindley, P., Pennock, J., Tomlinson, D., Weedon, D. and Carmichael, S. (1994) *Our Lifestyles: An Introductory Exercise for Anyone Meeting People with Learning Disabilities.* Brighton: Pavilion.

Brook Advisory Centre (1987) *Not A Child any more.* London: Brook Advisory Centres.

Brown, H. (1980) 'Sexual knowledge and education of ESN students in centres of further education.' *Sexuality and Disability 3,* 3, 215–220.

Brown, H. (1983) 'Why is it such a big secret?' In M. Craft and A. Craft (1983) *Sex Education and Counselling for Mentally Handicapped People.* Tunbridge Wells: Costello.

Brown, H. (1987) 'Working with parents.' In A. Craft (ed) *Mental Handicap and Sexuality: Issues and Perspectives.* Tunbridge Wells: Costello.

Brown, H. (1992) 'Working with staff around sexuality and power.' In A. Waitman and S. Conboy-Hill (eds) *Psychotherapy and Mental Handicap.* London: Sage.

Brown, H. (1993) 'Sexuality and intellectual disability: The new realism.' *Current Opinion in Psychiatry 6,* 623–628.

Brown, H. (1994) 'Lost in the system: Acknowledging the sexual abuse of adults with learning disabilities.' *Care In Place 1,* 2, 145–157.

Brown, H. Personal communication, 6.12.95.

Brown, H. (1996) 'Ordinary women: Issues for women with learning disabilities.' *British Journal of Learning Disabilities 24,* 47–51.

Brown, H. and Craft, A. (1992) *Working with the Unthinkable.* London: Family Planning Association.

Brown, H and Smith, H. (1989) 'Whose ordinary life is it anyway?' *Disability, Handicap and Society 4,* 2, 105–119.

Brown, H. and Smith, H. (1992) 'Assertion, not assimilation: A feminist perspective on the normalisation principle.' In H. Brown and H. Smith (eds) *Normalisation: A Reader for the Nineties.* London: Routledge.

Brown, H. and Stein, J. (eds) (1997a) *But Now They've Got a Voice: A Tape about Sexual Abuse for Service Users made by Service Users.* Brighton: Pavilion Publishing.

Brown, H. and Stein, J. (eds) (1997b) *A Nightmare that I Thought Would Never End: A Tape about Sexual Abuse for Staff made by Service Users.* Brighton: Pavilion Publishing.

Brown, H. and Turk, V. (1992) 'Defining sexual abuse as it affects adults with learning disabilities.' *Mental Handicap 20,* June, 44–55.

Brown, H., Hunt, N. and Stein, J. (1995) '"Alarming, but very necessary": Working with staff groups around the sexual abuse of adults with learning disabilities.' *Journal of Intellectual Disability Research 38,* 393–412.

Brown, H., Stein, J. and Turk, V. (1995) 'The sexual abuse of adults with learning disabilities: Report of a second two-year incidence survey.' *Mental Handicap Research 8,* 1, 3–24.

Brown, H. and Thompson, D. (1997) 'A minefield in a vacuum: The ethics of working with men with learning disabilities who have unacceptable or abusive sexual behaviours.' *Disability and Society 12,* 5, 695–707.

Brownmiller, S. (1976) *Against our Will: Men, Women and Rape.* London: Penguin.

Brownmiller, S. (1986) *Femininity.* London: Paladin.

Buchanan, A and Wilkins, R. (1991) 'Sexual abuse of the mentally handicapped: Difficulties in establishing prevalence.' *Psychiatric Bulletin 15,* 601–605.

Buck v. Bell. 274 U.S. 200 (1927) quoted by Justice Oliver Wendell Holmes. Cited in Craft, M and Craft, A. (1979) *Handicapped Married Couples.* London: Routledge and Kegan Paul.

Burchill, J. (1997) Death of innocence.' *The Guardian,* November 12th.

Burns, J. (1993) 'Invisible Women – Women who have learning difficulties.' *The Psychologist 6,* March, 102–105.

Burns, J. (1998) 'The functional use of sexuality by women with learning disabilities.' Paper given at Sexuality and Women with Learning Disabilities Conference, London, 7 July.

Burstow, B. (1992) *Radical Feminist Therapy: Working in the Context of Violence.* Newberry Park, California: Sage.

Bull, N. (1994) *Colour Me Loud.* A Mental Health Media Production for Channel Four.

Cambridge, P. (1995) *What You Need to Know about HIV and AIDS.* Kidderminster: BILD.

Cambridge, P. (1997) *HIV, Sex and Learning Disability.* Brighton: Pavilion Publishing.

Cambridge, P., Hayes, L., Knapp, M., Gould, E. and Fenyo, A. (1994) *Care in the Community: Five Years On.* Aldershot: Arena.

Cambridge, P., Beecham, J., Carbenlier, J. and Knapp, M. (1996) *Ten Years On: Outcomes and Costs of Community Care for People with Learning Disabilities and Mental Health Problems.* Research proposal to Dept. of Health. Canterbury: Tizard Centre/PSSRU.

Cambridge, P. and Brown, H. (1997) 'Making the market work for people with learning disabilities.' *Critical Social Policy 17,* 2, 27–52.

Cambridge, P. and McCarthy, M. (1997) 'Developing and implementing a sexuality policy for a learning disability provider service.' *Health and Social Care in the Community 5,* 3, 1–10.

Campbell, B. (1983) 'Sex – a family affair.' In L. Segal (ed) *What is to be Done about the Family? Crisis in the Eighties.* London: Penguin.

Campbell, B. (1988) *Unofficial Secrets. Child Sexual Abuse: The Cleveland Case.* London: Virago.

Carson, D. (1989) 'Why the law lords must rule on sterilization.' *Health Service Journal,* 9 March, 295.

Carson, D. (1994) 'The law's contribution to protecting people with learning disabilities from physical and sexual abuse.' In J. Harris and A. Craft (eds) *B.I.L.D. Seminar Papers No. 4: People with Learning Disabilities at Risk of Physical or Sexual Abuse.* Kidderminster: BILD.

Chamberlain, A., Rauh, J., Passer, A., McGrath, M. and Burket, R. (1984) 'Issues in fertility control for mentally retarded female adolescents: 1. Sexual activity, sexual abuse and contraception.' *Pediatrics, 73,* 4, 445–450.

Chenoweth, L. (1992) 'Invisible acts: Violence against women with disabilities.' *Australian Disability Review 2,* 22–27.

Chenoweth, L. (1996) 'Violence and women with disabilities: Silence and paradox.' *Violence Against Women 2,* 4, 391–411.

Churchill, J., Brown, H., Craft, A. and Horrocks, C. (eds) (1997) *There Are No Easy Answers.* Chesterfield and Nottingham: ARC/NAPSAC.

Clare, I. and Gudjonsson, G. (1991) 'Recall and understanding of the caution and rights in police detention among persons of average intellectual ability and persons with a mild mental handicap.' *Issues in Criminological and Legal Psychology 17,* 1, 34–42.

Clegg, S. (1985) 'Feminist methodology – Fact or fiction?' *Quality and Quantity 19,* 83–97.

Clements, J., Clare, I. and Ezelle, L. (1995) 'Real men, real women, real lives? Gender issues in learning disabilities and challenging behaviour.' *Disability and Society 10,* 4, 425–435.

Cocks, E. and Cockram, J. (1995) 'The participatory research paradigm and intellectual disability.' *Mental Handicap Research 8,* 1, 25–37.

Cohen, P. (1994) 'Bearing witness.' *Community Care,* 30 April, 20–21.

Collins, J. (1995) 'Moving forward or moving back? Institutional trends in services for people with learning difficulties.' In T. Philpot and L. Ward (eds) *Values and Visions: Changing Ideas in Services for People with Learning Difficulties.* Oxford: Butterworth- Heinemann.

Collins, J. (1997) 'Integration or sanctuary?' *Community Care,* 23–29 January, 29.

Colour Me Loud (1994) A Mental Health Media Production for Channel Four. A video about self-advocacy for people with learning disabilities.

Commissioners in Lunacy (1871) 25th Annual Report. Cited in A. Scull (1993) *The Most Solitary of Afflictions: Madness and Society in Britain 1700–1900.* New Haven and London: Yale University Press.

Copperman, J. amd Burrows, F. (1992) 'Reducing the risk of assault.' *Nursing Times 88,* 26, 64–65.

Cotterill, P. (1992) 'Interviewing women: Issues of friendship, vulnerability and power.' *Women's Studies International Forum 15,* 5/6, 593–606.

Craft, A. (1980) *Educating Mentally Handicapped People.* London: Camera Talks Ltd.

Craft, A. (1983a) 'Sexuality and mental retardation: A review of the literature.' In M. Craft and A. Craft (eds) *Sex Education and Counselling for Mentally Handicapped People.* Tunbridge Wells: Costello.

Craft, A. (1983b) 'Teaching programmes and training techniques.' In M. Craft and A. Craft (eds) *Sex Education and Counselling for Mentally Handicapped People.* Tunbridge Wells: Costello.

Craft, A. (1985) *Educating Mentally Handicapped People.* London: Camera Talks Ltd.

Craft, A. (1987) *Mental Handicap and Sexuality: Issues and Perspectives.* Tunbridge Wells: Costello.

Craft, A. (1992) 'Remedies for difficulties.' *Community Care,* 25 June, supplement iii – iv.

Craft, A. and members of the Nottinghamshire SLD sex education project. (1991) *Living Your Life.* Cambridge: Learning Development Aids.

Craft, A., Stewart, D., Mallett, A., Martin, D. and Tomlinson, S. (1996) 'Sex education for students with severe learning difficulties.' *Health Education 6,* 11–18.

Craft, M. and Craft, A. (1979) *Handicapped Married Couples*. London: Routledge and Kegan Paul.

Craft, M. and Craft, A. (1983) *Sex Education and Counselling for Mentally Handicapped People*. Tunbridge Wells: Costello.

Crawford, J., Kippax, S. and Waldby, C. (1994) 'Women's sex talk and men's sex talk: Different worlds.' *Feminism and Psychology 4*, 4, 571–587.

Crossmaker, M. (1991) 'Behind closed doors – Institutional sexual abuse.' *Sexuality and Disability 9*, 3, 210–219.

Dalley, G. (1988) *Ideologies of Caring: Rethinking Community and Collectivism*. Basingstoke: Macmillan Education.

d'Ardenne, P. and Mahtani, A. (1989) *Transcultural Counselling in Action*. London: Sage.

Daniels, A. (1967) 'The low-caste stranger in social research.' In G. Sjoberg (ed) *Ethics, Politics and Social Research*. Cambridge, MA: Schenkman.

Davies, A. (1978) 'Rape, racism and the capitalist setting.' *Black Scholar 9*, 7, 24–30.

Davies, N. (1998) 'The epidemic in our midst.' *The Guardian*, 2 June.

Davis, L. (1987) 'Who knows best?' *Nursing Times 84*, 4, 48.

Deegan, M. and Brooks, N. (1985) *Women and Disability: The Double Handicap*. New Brunswick: Transaction.

Demetral, G., Driessen, J. and Goff, G. (1983) 'A proactive training approach designed to assist developmentally disabled adolescents deal effectively with their menarche.' *Sexuality and Disability 6*, 1, 38–46.

Dept. of Health (1998) *Health and Personal Social Services Statistics for England*. London: Dept. of Health.

Dept. of Health and Social Security (1969) Report of the Committee of Enquiry into the Allegations of Ill Treatment and Other Irregularities at the Ely Hospital, Cardiff. Cmnd 3975, London: HMSO.

Dept. of Health and Home Office (1992) Review of Health and Social Services for Mentally Disordered Offenders and Others Requiring Similar Services. Final Report Summary (The Reed Committee Report). London: HMSO.

Dickson, A. (1985) *The Mirror Within*. London: Quartet Books.

Dixon, H. (1986) *Options for Change: A Staff Training Handbook on Personal Relationships and Sexuality for People with a Mental Handicap*. London: FPA Education Unit and B.I.M.H.

Dixon, H. (1988) *Sexuality and Mental Handicap*. Cambridge: Learning Development Aids.

Dobash, R. and Dobash, R. (1980) *Violence Against Wives*. London: Open Books.

Donnelly, M., McGilloway, S., Mays, N., Perry, S., Knapp, M., Kavanagh, S., Beecham, J., Fenyo, A. and Astin, J. (1994) *Opening New Doors: An Evaluation of Community Care for People Discharged from Psychiatric and Mental Handicap Hospitals*. London: HMSO.

Downes, M. (1982) 'Counselling women with developmental disabilities.' *Women and Therapy 1*, 3, 101–109.

Downs, C. and Craft, A. (1997) *Sex in Context*. Brighton: Pavilion Publishers.

Dumfries and Galloway Social Work Dept. (undated) 'The sexuality of people with a mental handicap: Policy and guidelines for staff working with mentally handicapped adults.'

Dunn, P. (1990) 'The impact of the housing environment upon the ability of disabled people to live independently.' *Disability, Handicap and Society 5*, 1, 37–52.

Dunne, J. and McLoone, J. (1988) 'The client terminology cycles.' In R. McConkey and P. McGinley (eds) *Concepts and Controversies in Services for People with Mental Handicap*. Galway and Dublin: Woodlands Centre and St. Michael's House.

Dunne, T. and Power, A. (1990) 'Sexual abuse and mental handicap: Preliminary findings from a community based study.' *Mental Handicap Research 3*, 111–125.

Dworkin, A. (1981) *Pornography: Men Possessing Women*. London: Women's Press.

Dworkin, A. (1987) *Intercourse*. London: Arrow Books.

East Sussex County Council (undated) 'Personal relationships and sexuality: Guidelines for carers working with people with learning disabilities.'

Edgerton, R. (1967) *The Cloak of Competence*. Berkeley: University of California Press.

Eisikovits, Z. and Buchbinder, E. (1997) 'A phenomenological study of metaphors battering men use.' *Violence Against Women 3*, 5, 482–498.

Elkins, T., Gatford, L., Wilks, C., Muram, D. and Golden, G. (1986) 'A model clinic for reproductive health concerns of the mentally handicapped.' *Obstetrics and Gynecology 68*, 2, 185–188.

Elkins, T. (1994) 'A model clinic approach for the reproductive health care of persons with developmental disabilities.' In Craft, A. (ed) *Practice Issues in Sexuality and Learning Disabilities*. London: Routledge.

Elliott, M. (1993) *Female Sexual Abuse of Children: The Ultimate Taboo*. Harlow: Longman.

Ellis, H. (1936) *Studies in the Psychology of Sex: Volume 1*. (New edition) New York: Random House.

Ellison, S., Parker, S. and Kitson, D. (1998) 'Health screening for women with learning disabilities: A study in Nottingham.' *NAPSAC Bulletin*, July, 11–13.

Emerson, E. (1992) 'What is normalisation?' In Brown, H. and Smith, H. (eds) *Normalisation: A Reader for the Nineties*. London: Routledge.

Emerson, E., McGill, P. and Mansell, J. (1994) *Severe Learning Disabilities and Challenging Behaviour: Designing High Quality Services*. London: Chapman Hall.

Fairbrother, P. (1983) 'The parents' viewpoint.' In M. Craft and A. Craft (1983) *Sex Education and Counselling for Mentally Handicapped People*. Tunbridge Wells: Costello.

Family Planning Association of New South Wales (1993) *Feeling Sexy, Feeling Safe*. Sex education video for people with learning disabilities.

Family Planning Association, Auckland (1997) *Four Stories: A Video about Personal Relationships for People with Intellectual Disabilities*.

Farberow, N. (1963) Introduction. In N. Farberow (ed) *Taboo Topics*. New York: Atherton Press.

Feminist Review (1987) *Sexuality: A Reader*. London: Virago.

Ferns, P. (1992) 'Promoting race equality through normalisation.' In H. Brown and H. Smith (eds) *Normalisation: A Reader for the Nineties*. London: Routledge.

Ferrarotti, F. (1981) 'On the autonomy of the biographical method.' In D. Bertaux (ed) *Biography and Society*. London: Sage.

Fielding, N. (1990) 'Time to adapt to disability.' *Roof 15*, May/June, 13.

Fielding, N. (1993) 'Ethnography.' In N. Gilbert (ed) *Researching Social Life*. London: Sage.

Finch, J. (1984) '"It's great to have someone to talk to": The ethics and politics of interviewing women.' In C. Bell and H. Roberts (eds) *Social Researching: Politics, Problems and Practice*. London: Routledge and Kegan Paul.

Finch, J. and Groves, D. (1983) *A Labour of Love: Women, Work and Caring*. London: Routledge and Kegan Paul.

Fine, M. (1988) 'Sexuality, schooling and adolescent females: The missing discourse of desire.' *Harvard Educational Review 58*, 1, 29–53.

Fisher, T. (undated) *Confessions of a Closet Sex Researcher*. Information leaflet from Society for the Scientific Study of Sex, P.O. Box 208, Mount Vernon, IA 52314, USA.

Fleet, M. and Johnston, P. (1996) 'Paedophile escapes on day trip.' *Daily Telegraph*, 31 August.

Flynn, M. (1986) 'Adults who are mentally handicapped as consumers: Issues and guidelines for interviewing.' *Journal of Mental Deficiency Research 30*, 369–377.

Foucault, M. (1990) *History of Sexuality: Volume 1, An Introduction*. London: Penguin.

Francis, J. (1996) 'Fight on all sides.' *Community Care*, 29 August, 12–13.

Fraser, J. and Ross, C. (1986) 'Time of the month.' *Nursing Times*, 2 July, 56–57.

Freud, S. (1979) *Civilisation and its Discontents*. London: Hogarth.

Friday, N. (1991) *Women On Top: How Real Life has Changed Women's Sexual Fantasies*. London: Hutchinson.

Friedan, B. (1963) *The Feminine Mystique*. New York: W.W.Norton Co.

Fruin, D. (1994) 'Almost equal opportunities… Developing personal relationship guidelines for social services department staff working with people with learning disabilities.' In A. Craft (ed) *Practice Issues in Sexuality and Learning Disabilities*. London: Routledge.

Gagnon, J. (1977) *Human Sexualities*. Glenview, IL: Scott, Foresman & Co.

Gagnon, J. and Simon, W. (1974) *Sexual Conduct: The Social Sources of Human Sexuality*. London: Hutchinson.

Gardiner, M., Kelly, K. and Wilkinson, D. (1996) 'Group for male sex offenders with learning disabilities.' *NAPSAC Bulletin*, March, 3–6.

Gath, A. (1988) 'Mentally handicapped people as parents.' *Journal of Child Psychology and Psychiatry 29*, 6, 739–744.

Gavey, N. (1992) 'Technologies and effects of heterosexual coercion.' *Feminism and Psychology 2*, 3, 325–351.

Gerrard, N. (1998) 'Uncharted territory.' *The Observer*, 16 August.

Goffman, E. (1961) *Asylums: Essays on the Social Situation of Mental Patients and Other Inmates*. New York: Doubleday.

Gordon, L. (1990) *Woman's Body, Woman's Right: Birth Control in America*. New York: Penguin Books.

Greengross, W. (1976) *Entitled to Love: The Sexual and Emotional Needs of the Handicapped*. London: Malaby Press Ltd.

Greenswag, L. (1987) 'Adults with Prader-Willi Syndrome: A survey of 232 cases.' *Developmental Medicine and Child Neurology 29*, 145–152.

Greenwich Social Services (undated) 'Recognising and responding to the abuse of adults with learning disabilities.'

Griffin, S. (1971) 'Rape: The all-American crime.' *Ramparts 10*, 3, 26–35.

Gudjonsson, G., Clare, I. and Cross, P. (1992) 'The revised PACE "Notice to detained persons": How easy is it to understand?' *Journal of the Forensic Science Society 32*, 289–299.

Hall, R. (1985) *Ask Any Woman*. Bristol: Falling Wall Press.

Hard, S. and Plumb, W. (1987) 'Sexual abuse of persons with developmental disabilities. A case study.' Unpublished manuscript.

Harding, S. (1987) *Feminism and Methodology*. Bloomington and Milton Keynes: Indiana University Press and Open University Press.

Hart, E. and Bond, M. (1995) *Action Research for Health and Social Care: A Guide to Practice*. Buckingham: Open University Press.

Hattersley, J., Hosking, G., Morrow, D. and Myers, M. (1987) *People with a Mental Handicap: Perspectives on Intellectual Disability*. London: Faber and Faber.

Hawkes, G. (1996) *A Sociology of Sex and Sexuality*. Buckingham: Open University Press.

Hazlehurst, M. (1993) *Breaking In, Breaking Out: Social and Sex Education for Men with Learning Disabilities.* London: Working With Men/The B Team.

Hepstinall, D. (1994) 'Sexual abuse: Justice means too many hurdles.' *Community Living,* April, 7–9.

Hertfordshire County Council Social Services Dept (1989) *Departmental Policies and Guidelines for Staff on the Sexual and Personal Relationships of People with a Mental Handicap.* Hertford: Hertfordshire County Council.

Heyman, B. and Huckle, S. (1995) 'Sexuality as a perceived hazard in the lives of adults with learning disabilities.' *Disability and Society 11,* 2, 139–155.

Hill Collins, P. (1991) *Black Feminist Thought: Knowledge, Consciousness and the Politics of Empowerment.* London: Routledge.

Hingsburger, D. (1987) 'Sex counselling with the developmentally handicapped: The assessment and management of seven critical problems.' *Psychiatric Aspects of Mental Retardation Reviews 6,* 9, 41–46.

Hingsburger, D. (1995) *Just Say Know!* Quebec: Diverse City Press.

Hingsburger, D. and Ludwig, S. (1992) 'Review of facts of life and living.' *SIECCAN Newsletter 27,* 2, 21–23.

Hite, S. (1976) *The Hite Report.* London: Pandora.

Hite, S. (1981) *The Hite Report on Male Sexuality.* London: Macdonald Optima.

Hite, S. (1988) *Women and Love.* London: Viking.

Holland, J., Ramazanoski, C., Scott, S., Sharpe, S. and Thomson, R. (1990) *'Don't Die of Ignorance'* – *I Nearly Died of Embarrassment. Condoms in Context.* WRAP Paper 2. London: Tufnell Press.

Holland, J., Ramazanoski, C., Scott, S., Sharpe, S. and Thomson, R. (1991a) *Pressure, Resistance, Empowerment: Young Women and the Negotiation of Safer Sex.* WRAP Paper 6. London: Tufnell Press.

Holland, J. Ramazanoski, C. and Sharpe, S. (1991b) *Pressured Pleasure: Young Women and the Negotiation of Sexual Boundaries.* WRAP Paper 7. London: Tufnell Press.

Holland, J. (1992) 'Risk, power and the possibility of pleasure: Young women and safer sex.' *AIDS Care 4,* 3, 273–283.

Holland, J., Ramazanoski, C. and Sharpe, S. (1993) *Wimp or Gladiator: Contradictions in Acquiring Masculine Sexuality.* WRAP/MRAP Paper 9. London: Tufnell Press.

Holland, J., Ramazanoski, C., Sharpe, S. and Thomson, R. (1998) *The Male in the Head: Young People, Heterosexuality and Power.* London: Tufnell Press.

Holland, J. and Ramazanoglu, C. (1994) 'Coming to conclusions: Power and interpretation in researching young women's sexuality.' In M. Maynard and J. Purvis (eds) *Researching Women's Lives From a Feminist Perspective.* London: Taylor and Francis.

Homan, R. (1991) *The Ethics of Social Research.* New York: Longman.

Home Office (1998) *Speaking Up for Justice: Report of the Interdepartmental Working Group on the Treatment of Vulnerable or Intimidated Witnesses in the Criminal Justice System.* London: Home Office.

hooks, b. (1984) *Feminist Theory: From Margin to Centre.* Boston: South End Press.

Horizon NHS Trust (1994) *Sexual Abuse Guidelines.*

Huovinen, K. (1996) 'Therapeutic ammenorrhea in mentally retarded women, at which age to stop?' *Trends in Biomedicine in Finland 7* (supplement), 58–61.

Hutchinson, P., Beechy, L., Foerster, C. and Fowlee, B. (1993) 'Double jeopardy: Women with disabilities speak out about community and relationships.' *Entourage 7,* 2, 16–18.

Itzin, C. (1994) *Pornography. Women, Violence and Civil Liberties: A Radical New View.* Oxford: Oxford University Press.

Jackson, M. (1983) 'Sexual liberation or social control?' *Women's Studies International Forum 6,* 1, 1–17.

Jackson, M. (1984) 'Sex research and the construction of sexuality: A tool of male supremacy?' *Women's Studies International Forum 7,* 1, 43–51.

Jackson, M. (1987) '"Facts of Life" or the eroticization of women's oppression? Sexology and the social construction of heterosexuality.' In P. Caplan (ed) *The Cultural Construction of Sexuality.* London: Routledge.

Jackson, M. (1994) *The Real Facts of Life: Feminism and the Politics of Sexuality c. 1850–1940.* London: Taylor and Francis.

Jackson, S. (1978) *On the Social Construction of Female Sexuality.* Explorations in Feminism Series, No. 4. London: Women's Research and Resources Centre Publications.

Jeffreys, S. (1984) '"Free from all uninvited touch of man": Women's campaigns around sexuality 1880–1914.' In L. Coveney, M. Jackson, S. Jeffreys, L. Kaye and P. Mahoney (eds) *The Sexuality Papers.* London: Hutchinson.

Jeffreys, S. (1985) 'Prostitution.' In D. Rhodes and S. MacNeil (eds) *Women Against Violence Against Women.* London: Onlywomen Press.

Jeffreys, S. (1990) *Anticlimax: A Feminist Perspective on the Sexual Revolution.* London: Women's Press.

Jeffreys, S. (1994) *The Lesbian Heresy: A Feminist Perspective on the Lesbian Sexual Revolution.* London: The Woman's Press.

Jensen, R. (1996) 'Knowing pornography.' *Violence Against Women 2,* 1, 82–102.

Johnson, P. and Davies, R. (1989) 'Sexual attitudes of members of staff.' *British Journal of Mental Subnormality 35,* 1, 17–21.

Jones, J. (1991) 'Street health work with men who cottage.' In *Health Education Authority Outreach Work with Men who Have Sex with Men.* London: Health Education Authority.

Kaeser, F. (1992) 'Can people with severe mental retardation consent to mutual sex?' *Sexuality and Disability 10,* 1, 33–42.

Katz, G. (undated) *Sexual Rights of the Retarded: Two Papers Reflecting the International Point of View.* London: National Association for Mentally Handicapped Children.

Kelly, L. (1988) *Surviving Sexual Violence.* Cambridge: Polity Press.

Kelly, L. (1996) '"When does the speaking profit us?": Reflections on the challenges of developing feminist perspectives on abuse and violence by women.' In M. Hester, L. Kelly and J. Radford (eds) *Women, Violence and Male Power.* Buckingham: Open University Press.

Kempton, W. (1972) *Guidelines for Planning a Training Course on Human Sexuality and the Retarded.* Philadelphia: Planned Parenthood Association of Southern Pennsylvania.

Kempton, W. (1988) *Life Horizons I and II.* Santa Monica: James Stanfield and Co.

Kempton, W., Bass, M. and Gordon, S. (1971) *Love, Sex and Birth Control for the Mentally Retarded: A Guide for Parents.* Philadelphia: Planned Parenthood Association of Southern Pennsylvania.

Kempton, W. and Kahn, E. (1991) 'Sexuality and people with intellectual disabilities: A historical perspective.' *Sexuality and Disability 9,* 2, 93–111.

Kennedy Bergen, R. (1993) 'Interviewing survivors of marital rape: Doing feminist research on sensitive topics.' In C. Renzetti and R. Lee (eds) *Researching Sensitive Topics.* London: Sage.

Khanna, S. and Kapur, R. (1996) *Memorandum on Reform of Laws Relating to Sexual Offences.* New Delhi: Centre for Feminist Legal Research.

Kiehlbauch Cruz, V., Price-Williams, D. and Andron, L. (1988) 'Developmentally disabled women who were molested as children.' *Social Casework: The Journal of Social Work,* September, 411–419.

Kinsey, A., Pomeroy, W. and Martin, C. (1948) *Sexual Behaviour in the Human Male.* Philadelphia: W.B.Saunders.

Kinsey, A., Pomeroy, W., Martin, C. and Gebhard, P. (1953) *Sexual Behaviour in the Human Female.* Philadelphia: W.B.Saunders.

Knapp, M., Cambridge, P., Thomason, C., Beecham, J., Allen, C. and Davton, C. (1992) *Care in the Community: Challenge and Demonstration.* Aldershot: Ashgate.

Koedt, A. (1970) 'The myth of the vaginal orgasm.' In L. Tanner (ed) *Voices from Women's Liberation.* New York: Signet Books.

Koegel, P. and Whittemore, R. (1983) 'Sexuality in the ongoing lives of mildly retarded adults.' In A. Craft and M. Craft (eds) *Sex Education and Counselling for Mentally Handicapped People.* Tunbridge Wells: Costello.

Korman, N. and Glennerster, H. (1990) *Hospital Closure: A Political and Economic Study.* Milton Keynes: Open University Press.

Krajicek, M. (1982) 'Developmental disability and human sexuality: Symposium on sexuality and nursing practice.' *Nursing Clinics of North America 17,* 3, 377–386.

Labour Research (1992) 'Outlawing disability bias.' *Labour Research 8,* 17–18.

Landman, R. (1994) *Let's Talk About Sex? Accessing Sex Education Services for Black People with Learning Difficulties.* Birmingham: East Birmingham Health Promotion Service.

Laslett, P. (1965) *The World We Have Lost.* London: Methuen.

Law Commission (1995) *Mental Incapacity.* Law Com. No. 231. London: HMSO.

Lawrence, M. (1987) Introduction. In M. Lawrence (ed) *Fed Up and Hungry: Women, Oppression and Food.* London: Women's Press.

Laws, S. (1990) *Issues of Blood: The Politics of Menstruation.* Basingstoke: Macmillan.

Lee, G. (1972) *Sexual Rights of the Retarded: Two Papers Reflecting the International Point of View.* London: National Association for Mentally Handicapped Children.

Lee, J. (1996) 'Addressing the issues relating to the sexuality of people with learning disabilities.' *Irish Journal of Occupational Therapy 26,* 1, 13–17.

Lee, R. (1993) *Doing Research on Sensitive Topics.* London: Sage.

Lees, S. (1993) *Sugar and Spice: Sexuality and Adolescent Girls.* London: Penguin.

Lees, S. (1996) *Carnal Knowledge: Rape on Trial.* London: Hamish Hamilton.

Lees, S. (1997) *Ruling Passions: Sexual Violence, Reputations and the Law.* Buckingham: Open University Press.

Lewisham Social Services (1992) *Take Care of Yourself Posters.* London: Lewisham HIV, Drugs and Alcohol Unit.

Leyin, A. and Dicks, M. (1987) 'Assessment and evaluation: Assessing what we are doing.' In A. Craft (ed) *Mental Handicap and Sexuality: Issues and Perspectives.* Tunbridge Wells: Costello.

Liazos, A. (1972) 'The poverty of the sociology of deviance: Nuts, sluts and perverts.' *Social Problems 20,* 102–120.

Lobel, K. (1986) *Naming the Violence: Speaking Out about Lesbian Battering.* Seattle: The Seal Press.

London Rape Crisis Centre (1988) *Sexual Violence: The Reality for Women.* London: Women's Press.

Lowes, L. (1977) *Sex and Social Training: A Programme for Young Adults.* London: National Association for Mentally Handicapped Children.

MacLeod, S. (1981) *The Art of Starvation.* London: Virago.

McCarthy, M. (1991) '"I don't mind sex, it's what the men do to you": Women with learning difficulties talking about their sexual experiences.' Unpublished MA dissertation, Middlesex Polytechnic.

McCarthy, M. (1993) 'Sexual experiences of women with learning difficulties in long-stay hospitals.' *Sexuality and Disability 11*, 4, 277–286.

McCarthy, M. (1994) 'Against all odds: HIV and safer sex education for women with learning difficulties.' In L. Doyal, J. Naidoo and T. Wilton (eds) *AIDS: Setting a Feminist Agenda*. London: Taylor and Francis.

McCarthy, M. (1995) 'Research into the sexuality of people with learning difficulties.' Paper presented at 'Research for Practitioners Seminar', Camden and Islington Health Authority, London, 21 September.

McCarthy, M. (1996a) 'Sexual experiences and sexual abuse of women with learning disabilities.' In M. Hester, L. Kelly and J. Radford (eds) *Women, Violence and Male Power*. Buckingham: Open University Press.

McCarthy, M. (1996b) 'The sexual support needs of people with learning disabilities: A profile of those referred for sex education.' *Sexuality and Disability 14*, 4, 265–279.

McCarthy, M. (1997) 'HIV and heterosexual sex.' In P. Cambridge and H. Brown (eds) *HIV and Learning Disability*. Kidderminster: BILD Publications.

McCarthy, M. (1998a) 'Whose body is it anyway?' *Disability and Society 13*, 4, 557–574.

McCarthy, M. (1998b) 'Sexual violence against women with learning disabilities.' *Feminism and Psychology 8*, 4, 544–551.

McCarthy, M. and Thompson, D. (1992) *Sex and the 3R's: Rights, Responsibilities and Risks*. Brighton: Pavilion.

McCarthy, M. and Thompson, D. (1994a) 'HIV/AIDS and safer sex work with people with learning disabilities.' In A. Craft (ed) *Practice Issues in Sexuality and Learning Disabilities*. London: Routledge.

McCarthy, M. and Thompson, D. (1994b) *Sex and Staff Training*. Brighton: Pavilion.

McCarthy, M. and Thompson, D. (1995) 'No more double standards: Sexuality and people with learning difficulties.' In T. Philpot and L. Ward (eds) *Values and Visions: Changing Ideas in Services for People with Learning Difficulties*. Oxford: Butterworth- Heinemann.

McCarthy, M. and Thompson, D. (1996) 'Sexual abuse by design: An examination of the issues in learning disability services.' *Disability and Society 11*, 2, 205–217.

McCarthy, M. and Thompson, D. (1997) 'A prevalence study of sexual abuse of adults with intellectual disabilities referred for sex education.' *Journal of Applied Research in Intellectual Disability 10*, 2, 105–124.

McCarthy, M. and Thompson, D. (1998) *Sex and the 3R's: Rights, Responsibilities and Risks – Second Edition*. Brighton: Pavilion.

MacIntyre, A. (1982) 'Risk, harm and benefit assessments as instruments of moral evaluation.' In T. Beauchamp, R. Faden, R. Wallace and L. Walters (eds) *Ethical Issues in Social Science Research*. Baltimore: Johns Hopkins University Press.

McKiernan, J. and McWilliams, M. (1994) 'Domestic violence in a violent society: The implications for abused women and children.' *Rights of Women Bulletin*, Spring, 13–19.

MacKinnon, C. (1987) 'Feminism, marxism, method and the state: Towards feminist jurisprudence.' In S. Harding (1987) *Feminism and Methodology*. Bloomington and Milton Keynes: Indiana University Press and Open University Press.

McLeod, J. (1994) *Doing Counselling Research*. London: Sage.

McSherry, B. (1998) 'Sexual assault against individuals with mental impairment: Are criminal laws adequate?' *Psychiatry, Psychology and Law 5*, 1, 107–116.

McNeil, S. (1985) 'In steering women who have been raped to sex therapists we are performing a function for men, and gluing over a crack in male supremacy.' In D. Rhodes and S. McNeil (eds) *Women Against Women Against Women*. London: Onlywomen Press.

Malinowski, B. (1950) *Argonauts of the Western Pacific*. New York: Dutton.

Malhotra, S. and Mellan, B. (1996) 'Cultural and race issues in sexuality work with people with learning difficulties.' *Tizard Learning Disability Review 1*, 4, 7–12.

Mama, A. (1986) 'Black women and the economic crisis.' In Feminist Review (eds) *Waged Work*. London: Virago.

Mama, A. (1989) *The Hidden Struggle: Statutory and Voluntary Sector Responses to Violence against Black Women in the Home*. London: London Race and Housing Research Unit.

Mansell, J. and Ericcson, K. (1996) *Deinstitutionalization and Community Living: Intellectual disability services in Britain, Scandinavia and the USA*. London: Chapman & Hall.

Marchant, C. (1993a) 'Protect and survive.' *Community Care*, 30 December, 12–13.

Marchant, C. (1993b) 'A need to know issue.' *Community Care*, 28 October, 11.

Matthews, H. (1994) 'What staff need to know.' *It Did Happen Here: Sexual Abuse and Learning Disability Conference Proceedings*. London: St. George's Mental Health Library Conference Series.

Mattinson, J. (1970) *Marriage and Mental Handicap*. London: Duckworth.

Maynard, M. (1994) 'Methods, practice and epistemology: The debate about feminism and research.' In M. Maynard and J. Purvis (eds) *Researching Women's Lives From a Feminist Perspective*. London: Taylor and Francis.

Meade, W. (1993) 'Let's get down to oral sex.' *Cosmopolitan 88*, February, 142–143.

Mencap Homes Foundation (1987) *Staff Guidelines on Personal and Sexual Relationships of People with a Mental Handicap*. London: Mencap.

Millard, L. (1994) 'Between ourselves: Experiences of a women's group on sexuality and sexual abuse.' In A. Craft (ed) *Practice Issues in Sexuality and Learning Disabilities*. London: Routledge.

Miller, W. and Crabtree, B. (1992) 'Primary care research: A multimethod typology and qualitative road map.' In B. Crabtree and W. Miller (eds) *Doing Qualitative Research*. London: Sage.

Minkes, J., Townsley, R., Weston, C. and Williams, C. (1995) 'Having a voice: Involving people with learning difficulties in research.' *British Journal of Learning Disabilities 23*, 94–97.

Mitchell, L. (1987) 'Intervention in the inappropriate sexual behaviour of individuals with mental handicaps.' In A. Craft (ed) *Mental Handicap and Sexuality: Issues and Perspectives*. Tunbridge Wells: Costello.

Monat-Haller, R. (1992) *Understanding and Expressing Sexuality: Responsible Choices for Individuals with Developmental Disabilities*. Baltimore: Paul H. Brookes Publishing.

Money, J. (1988) 'Commentary: Current status of sex research.' *Journal of Psychology and Human Sexuality 1*, 6.

Monto, M. (1998) 'Holding men accountable for prostitution: The unique approach of the Sexual Exploitation Education Project.' *Violence Against Women 4*, 4, 505–517.

Moore, S. and Rosenthal, D. (1993) *Sexuality in Adolescence*. London: Routledge.

Moran-Ellis, J. (1996) 'Close to home: The experience of researching child sexual abuse.' In M. Hester, L. Kelly and J. Radford (eds) *Women, Violence and Male Power*. Buckingham: Open University Press.

Morris, J. (1992) 'Personal and political: A feminist perspective on researching physical disability.' *Disability, Handicap and Society* 7, 2, 157–166.

Morris, J. (ed) (1996) *Encounters with Strangers: Feminism and Disability.* London: Women's Press.

Morris, J. (1991) '"Us" and "them"? Feminist research, community care and disability.' *Critical Social Policy 11*, 3, 22–39.

Morris, P. (1969) *Put Away: A Sociological Study of Institutions for the Mentally Retarded.* London: Routledge and Kegan Paul.

Namdarkhan, L. (1995) 'Women with learning disabilities: Mixed sex living – Who benefits?' Unpublished MA Dissertation, Middlesex University.

Nirje, B. (1980) 'The normalisation principle.' In R. Flynn and K. Nitsch (eds) *Normalisation, Social Integration and Community Services.* Austin, TX: Pro-Ed.

Noonan Walsh, P. (1988) 'Handicapped and female: Two disabilities?' In R. McConkey and P. McGinley (eds) *Concepts and Controversies in Services for People with Mental Handicap.* Galway and Dublin: Woodlands Centre and St. Michael's House.

Oakley, A. (1981) 'Interviewing women: A contradiction in terms?' In H. Roberts (ed) *Doing Feminist Research.* London: Routledge and Kegan Paul.

O'Connor, W. (1996) 'A problem-solving intervention for sex offenders with an intellectual disability.' *Journal of Intellectual and Developmental Disability 21*, 3, 219–236.

Oliver, M. (1990) *The Politics of Disablement.* Basingstoke: Macmillan.

Oliver, M. (1992) 'Changing the social relations of research production?' *Disability, Handicap and Society* 7, 2, 101–114.

Orbach, S. (1978) *Fat Is A Feminist Issue.* New York and London: Paddington Press.

Orlando, J. and Koss, M. (1983) 'The effect of sexual victimisation on sexual satisfaction: A study of the negative-association hypothesis.' *Journal of Abnormal Psychology 92*, 1, 104–106.

O'Sullivan, A. and Gillies, P. (1993) *You, Me and HIV – Making Sense of Safer Sex.* Cambridge: Daniels Publishing.

Park, P. (1978) *Social Research and Radical Change.* Amherst: University of Massachusetts.

Pateman, C. (1980) 'Women and consent.' *Political Theory 8*, 2, 149–168.

People First (1991) *Policy Statement by Women with Learning Disabilities.* London: People First.

People First (undated) *Everything You Ever Wanted to Know about Safer Sex. . . but Nobody Bothered to Tell You.* London: People First.

People First (undated) *Women First: A Book by Women with Learning Difficulties about the Issues for Women with Learning Difficulties.* London: People First.

Petras, J. (1973) *Sexuality in Society.* Boston: Allyn and Bacon Inc.

Phoenix, A. (1994) 'Practising feminist research: The intersection of gender and "race" in the research process.' In M. Maynard and J. Purvis (eds) *Researching Women's Lives from a Feminist Perspective.* London: Taylor and Francis.

Phillips, A. and Rakusen, J. (1989) *Our Bodies, Ourselves: A Handbook by and for Women (British Edition).* London: Penguin.

Pizzey, E. (1974) *Scream Quietly or the Neighbours Will Hear.* Harmondsworth: Penguin.

Plummer, K. (1982) 'Symbolic interactionism and sexual conduct: An emergent perspective.' In M. Brake (ed) *Human Sexual Relations: Towards a Redefinition of Sexual Politics.* New York: Pantheon.

Plummer, K. (1995) *Telling Sexual Stories: Power, Change and Social Worlds.* London: Routledge.

Porter, R. (1982) 'Mixed feelings: The Enlightenment and sexuality in eighteenth century Britain.' In P. Bouce (ed) *Sexuality in Eighteenth Century Britain.* Manchester: Manchester University Press.

Potts, M. and Fido, R. (1991) *A Fit Person To Be Removed: Personal Accounts of Life in a Mental Deficiency Hospital.* Plymouth: Northcote House Publishers.

Powerhouse (1996a) 'Power in the house: Women with learning difficulties organising against abuse.' In J. Morris (ed) *Encounters with Strangers: Feminism and Disability.* London: Women's Press.

Powerhouse (1996b) 'What women from Powerhouse say about sexual abuse.' *Tizard Learning Disability Review 1,* 4, 39–43.

Quilliam, S. (1994) *Women On Sex.* London: Quality Paperbacks Direct (by arrangement with Smith Gryphon Ltd.).

Radford, J. and Stanko, E. (1996) 'Violence against women and children: The contradictions of crime control under patriarchy.' In M. Hester, L. Kelly and J. Radford (eds) *Women, Violence and Male Power.* Buckingham: Open University Press.

Ramazanoglu, C. (1992) 'Love and the politics of heterosexuality.' *Feminism and Psychology 2,* 3, 444–447.

Randall, M. and Haskell, L. (1995) 'Sexual violence in women's lives: Findings from the Women's Safety Project, a community based study.' *Violence Against Women 1,* 1, 6–31.

Rapley, M. and Antaki, C. (1996) 'A conversation analysis of the "acquiescence" of people with learning disabilities.' *Journal of Community and Applied Social Psychology 6,* 3, 207–227.

Ravaud, J., Madiot, B. and Ville, I. (1992) 'Discrimination towards disabled people seeking employment.' *Social Science and Medicine 35,* 8, 951–958.

Rees, S. and Berchert, R. (1992) 'An educational programme on HIV infection for formerly institutionalised people with developmental disabilities.' In A. Crocker, H. Cohen and T. Kastner (eds) *HIV Infection and Developmental Disabilities.* Baltimore: Paul H. Brookes Publishers.

Reich, W. (1969) *The Sexual Revolution: Toward a Self-Governing Character Structure.* 4th (revised) edition. New York: Farrar, Straus and Giroux.

Reinharz, S. (1983) 'Experiential analysis: A contribution to feminist research.' In G. Bowles and R. Duelli-Klein (eds) *Theories of Women's Studies.* Boston: Routledge and Kegan Paul.

Renshaw, J., Hampson, R., Thomason, C., Darton, C., Judge, K. and Knapp, M. (1988) *Care in the Community: The First Steps.* Aldershot: Gower Publishing Co.

Renzetti, C. and Lee, R. (1993) 'The problems of researching sensitive topics: An overview and introduction.' In C. Renzetti and R. Lee (eds) *Researching Sensitive Topics.* London: Sage Publications.

Rich, A. (1980) 'Compulsory heterosexuality and lesbian existence.' *Signs 5,* 4, 631–660.

Robb, B. (1967) *Sans Everything: A Case to Answer.* London: Nelson.

Robinson, S. (1987) 'Experiences of sex education programmes for adults who are intellectually handicapped.' In A. Craft (ed) *Mental Handicap and Sexuality: Issues and Perspectives.* Tunbridge Wells: Costello.

Rodgers, J. and Russell, O. (1995) 'Healthy lives: The health needs of people with learning difficulties.' In T. Philpot and L. Ward (eds) *Values and Visions: Changing Ideas in Services for People with Learning Difficulties.* Oxford: Butterworth-Heinemann.

Rose, H. (1982) 'Making science feminist.' In E. Whitelegg, M. Arnot, E. Barrels, V. Beechy, L. Birke, S. Himmelwert, D. Leonard, S. Ruehl and V. Speakman (eds) *The Changing Experience of Women.* Oxford: Blackwell, in association with Open University.

Rose, J. (1990) 'Accepting and developing the sexuality of people with mental handicaps: Working with parents.' *Mental Handicap 18*, March, 4–6.

Rose, J. and Jones, C. (1994) 'Working with parents.' In A. Craft (ed) *Practice Issues in Sexuality and Learning Disabilities*. London: Routledge.

Rosen, M. (1972) 'Psychosexual adjustment of the mentally handicapped.' In M. Bass and M. Gelof (eds) *Sexual Rights and Responsibilities of the Mentally Retarded*. Proceedings of the conference of American Association on Mental Deficiency, Region X.

Roseneil, S. (1993) 'Greenham revisited: Researching myself and my sisters.' In D. Hobbs and T. May (eds) *Interpreting the Field: Accounts of Ethnography*. Oxford: Oxford University Press.

Rosser, K. (1990) 'A particular vulnerability.' *Australian Legal Services Bulletin 15*, 1, 32–34.

Roy, M and Roy, A. (1988) 'Sterilization for girls and women with mental handicaps: Some ethical and moral considerations.' *Mental Handicap 16*, September, 97–100.

Russell, D. (1984) *'Sexual Exploitation: Rape, Child Sexual Abuse and Workplace Harassment.'* London: Sage.

Russell, D. (1995) 'The making of a whore.' *Violence Against Women 1*, 1, 77–98.

Ryan, M. (1993) 'Sex education for people with learning difficulties: Issues for parents.' In B. Mellan, M. McCarthy and M. Rooney (eds) *Sexuality and People with Learning Difficulties: Seminar Papers on Current Practice*. London: NWTRHA Publications.

Ryan, J. and Thomas, F. (1987) *The Politics of Mental Handicap*. Revised edition. London: Free Association Books.

Scally, B. (1973) 'Marriage and mental handicap: Some observations in Northern Ireland.' In F. de la Cruz and G. Laveck (eds) *Human Sexuality and the Mentally Retarded*. New York: Brunner/Mazel.

Schaefer, L. (1973) *Women and Sex*. London: Hutchinson.

Scott, L. and the Image in Action Team (1994) *On The Agenda*. London: Image In Action.

Scull, A. (1979) *Museums of Madness: The Social Organisation of Insanity in Nineteenth Century England*. London: Allen Lane.

Scull, A. (1993) *The Most Solitary of Afflictions: Madness and Society in Britain 1700–1900*. New Haven and London: Yale University Press.

Segal, L. (1983) 'Sensual uncertainty, or why the clitoris is not enough.' In S. Cartledge and J. Ryan (eds) *Sex and Love*. London: Women's Press.

Segal, L. (1987) *Is the Future Female? Troubled Thoughts on Contemporary Feminism*. London: Virago.

Segal, L. (1990) *Slow Motion: Changing Masculinities, Changing Men*. London: Virago.

Segal, L. (1994) *Straight Sex: The Politics of Pleasure*. London: Virago.

Segal, L. and McIntosh, M. (1992) *Sex Exposed: Sexuality and the Pornography Debate*. London: Virago.

Sgroi, S. (1989) 'Evaluation and treatment of sexual offence behaviour in persons with mental retardation.' In S. Sgroi (ed) *Vulnerable Populations*. Toronto: Lexington Books.

Shearer, A. (1986) *Building Community: With People with Mental Handicaps, their Families and Friends*. London: Campaign for People with Mental Handicaps and Kings Fund Publishing Office.

Sieber, J. and Stanley, B. (1988) 'Ethical and professional dimensions of socially sensitive research.' *American Psychologist 43*, 49–55.

Sigelman, C., Budd, E., Spenhel, C. and Schoenrock, C. (1981a) 'Asking questions of retarded persons: A comparison of yes-no and either-or formats.' *Applied Research in Mental Retardation 4*, 347–357.

Sigelman, C. Budd, E., Spenhel, C. and Schoenrock, C. (1981b) 'When in doubt, say yes: Acquiescence in interviews with mentally retarded persons.' *Mental Retardation 19*, 53–58.

Silverman, D. (1993) *Interpreting Qualitative Data: Methods for Analysing Talk, Text and Interaction.* London: Sage Publications.

Simons, K. (1992) *'Sticking Up for Yourself': Self-Advocacy and People with Learning Disabilities.* York: Joseph Rowntree Foundation.

Simons, K., Booth, T. and Booth, W. (1989) 'Speaking out: User studies and people with learning difficulties.' *Research, Policy and Planning 7*, 1, 9–17.

Simpson, D. (1994) *Sexual Abuse and People with Learning Difficulties: Developing Access to Community Services.* London: Family Planning Association.

Sinason, V. (1994) 'Working with sexually abused individuals who have a learning disability.' In A. Craft (ed) *Practice Issues in Sexuality and Learning Disabilities.* London: Routledge.

Skills for People (1994) *How to Run Courses in Self Advocacy for People with Learning Disabilities.* Brighton: Pavilion.

Smyth, C. (1992) *Lesbians Talk Queer Notions.* London: Scarlett Press.

Sobsey, D. (1994) *Violence and Abuse in the Lives of People with Disabilities: The End of Silent Acceptance?* Baltimore: Paul H. Brookes Publishing.

Sone, K. (1995) 'Lack of conviction?' *Community Care*, 8–14 June, 22–23.

South East London Health Promotion Services (1992) *My Choice, My Own Choice.* A sex education video for people with learning disabilities.

Spender, D. (1981) 'The gatekeepers: A feminist critique of academic publishing.' In Roberts, H. (ed) *Doing Feminist Research.* London: Routledge and Kegan Paul.

Spender, D. (1993) Preface. To S. Hite, *Women as Revolutionary Agents of Change: The Hite Reports 1972–93.* London: Bloomsbury.

Spradley, J. (1979) *The Ethnographic Interview.* New York: Holt, Rinehart and Winston.

Squire, J. (1989) 'Sex education for pupils with severe learning difficulties.' *Mental Handicap 17*, 66–69.

Stalker, K. (1998) 'Some ethical and methodological issues in research with people with learning difficulties.' *Disability and Society 13*, 1, 5–19.

Stanko, E. (1985) *Intimate Intrusions: Women's Experience of Male Violence.* London: Routledge and Kegan Paul.

Stanley, L. (1990) *Feminist Praxis: Research, Theory and Epistemology in Feminist Sociology.* London: Routledge.

Stanley, L. (1995) *Sex Surveyed 1949–1994: From Mass Observation's 'Little Kinsey' to the National Survey and the Hite Reports.* London: Taylor and Francis.

Stanley, L. and Wise, S. (1993) *Breaking Out Again: Feminist Ontology and Epistemology.* London: Routledge.

Stenfert Kroese, B., Gillot, A. and Atkinson, V. (1998) 'Consumers with intellectual disabilities as service evaluators.' *Journal of Applied Research in Intellectual Disability 11*, 2, 116–128.

Stevens, P. (1994) 'Protective strategies of lesbian clients in health care environments.' *Research in Nursing and Health 17*, 217–229.

Stevens, S., Evered, C., O'Brien, R. and Wallace, G. (1988) 'Sex education: Who needs it?' *Mental Handicap 16*, 166–170.

Stewart, D. (1993) 'Sex education for young people with learning difficulties in a school setting.' In Mellan, B., M. McCarthy, M. Rooney (eds) *Sexuality and People with Learning Difficulties: Seminar Papers on Current Practice.* London: NWTRHA Publications.

Stewart, M. (1981) 'Sexual intercourse and system maintenance in feminist perspective.' *Free Inquiry in Creative Sociology 9*, 2, 165–181.

Stewart, W. (1979) *The Sexual Side of Handicap: A Guide for the Caring Professions.* Cambridge: Woodhead-Faulkner.

Stewart, W. (1995) *Cassell's Queer Companion: A Dictionary of Lesbian and Gay Life and Culture.* London: Cassell.

Stromsness, M. (1993) 'Sexually abused women with mental retardation: Hidden victims, absent resources.' *Women and Therapy 14*, 3–4, 139–152.

Swain, J., Heyman, B. and Gillman, M. (1998) 'Public research, private concerns: Ethical issues in the use of open-ended interviews with people who have learning difficulties.' *Disability and Society 13*, 1, 21–36.

Szekely, E. (1988) *Never Too Thin.* Toronto: The Women's Press.

Szasz, T. (1980) *Sex: Facts, Frauds and Follies.* Oxford: Basil Blackwell.

Tate, T. (1998) 'They abused children (but only for research purposes).' *The Observer,* 9 August.

Taylor, M. and Carlson, G. (1993) 'The legal trends: Implications for menstruation/ fertility management for young women who have an intellectual disability.' *International Journal of Disability, Development and Education 40*, 2, 133–157.

Thaler Green, D. (1983) 'A human sexuality programme for developmentally disabled women in a sheltered workshop setting.' *Sexuality and Disability 6*, 1, 20–24.

Thompson, D. (1993) *Learning Disabilities: The Fundamental Facts.* London: Mental Health Foundation.

Thompson, D. (1994a) 'The sexual experiences of men with learning disabilities having sex with men: Issues of HIV prevention.' *Sexuality and Disability 12*, 3, 221–242.

Thompson, D. (1994b) 'Sexual experience and sexual identity for men with learning disabilities who have sex with men.' *Changes 12*, 4, 254–263.

Thompson, D. (1995) 'HIV and People with learning disabilities: Difficult questions, time for answers.' *Health Psychology Update 19*, 14–18.

Thompson, D. (1997) 'Profiling the sexually abusive behaviour of men with learning disabilities.' *Journal of Applied Research in Intellectual Disability 10*, 2, 125– 139.

Thompson, D. (1998) 'The Sexual Experiences and Sexual Identity of Men with Learning Disabilities.' Unpublished PhD manuscript, University of Kent.

Thompson, D. Personal communication, 24.8.98.

Thompson, D., Clare, I. and Brown, H. (1997) 'Not such an "ordinary" relationship: The role of women support staff in relation to men with learning disabilities who have difficult sexual behaviour.' *Disability and Society 12*, 4, 573–592.

Thompson, D. and Brown, H. (1998) *Response-ability.* Brighton: Pavilion.

Thomson, R. (1994) 'Moral rhetoric and public health pragmatism: The recent politics of sex education.' *Feminist Review 48*, Autumn, 40–60.

Thomson, R. and Scott, S. (1991) *Learning about Sex: Young Women and the Social Construction of Sexual Identity.* WRAP Paper 4. London: Tufnell Press.

Tonkin, B. (1987) 'Under a cloak of silence.' *Community Care,* 30 April, 18–19.

Thompson, S. (1990) 'Putting a big thing into a little hole: Teenage girls accounts of sexual initiation.' *Journal of Sex Research 27*, 3, 341–361.

Tiefer, L. (1995) *Sex Is Not a Natural Act.* Boulder, Colorado: Westview Press.

Townsend, P. (1962) *The Last Refuge: A Survey of Residential Institutions and Homes for the Aged in England and Wales.* London: Routledge and Kegan Paul.

Townsley, R. (1995) 'Avon calling.' *Community Care*, 12–18 January, 26–27.

Trent, J. (1994) *Inventing the Feeble Mind: A History of Mental Retardation in the United States*. Berkeley and Los Angeles: University of California Press.

Troiden, R. (1987) 'Walking the line: The personal and professional risks of sex education and research.' *Teaching Sociology 15*, 241–249.

Tuke, S. (1813) *Description of the Retreat, An Institution near York, for Insane Persons of the Society of Friends*. York: W. Alexander.

Turner, S. (1996) 'Healthy bodies, healthy minds.' *Community Care* 5–10 January, 24–25.

Tymchuk, A., Andron, L and Unger, O. (1987) 'Parents with mental handicaps and adequate childcare – a review.' *Mental Handicap 15*, 49–53.

Van Zijderfeld, B. (1987) 'Personal relationships and sex education – The Dutch experience.' In A. Craft (ed) *Mental Handicap and Sexuality: Issues and Perspectives*. Tunbridge Wells: Costello.

Vance, C. (1983) 'Gender systems, ideology and sex research.' In A. Snitow, C. Stansell and S. Thompson (eds) *Powers of Desire: The Politics of Sexuality*. New York: Monthly Review Press.

Walmsley, J. (1993) 'Women First: Lessons in participation.' *Critical Social Policy 13*, 2, 86–99.

Walsall Women's Group (1994) *No Means No*. Walsall: Learning For Living Scheme.

Ward, E. (1984) *Father–Daughter Rape*. London: Women's Press.

Weber, M. (1947) *The Theory of Economic and Social Organisation*. Glencoe, IL: The Free Press.

Weeks, J. (1985) *Sexuality and its Discontents – Meanings, Myths and Modern Sexualities*. London: Routledge.

Weeks, J. (1986) *Sexuality*. Chichester: Ellis Horwood Ltd.

Weeks, J. (1989b) *Sex, Politics and Society: The Regulation of Sexuality since 1800*. London: Longman.

Weeks, J. (1991) *Against Nature: Essays on History, Sexuality and Identity*. London: Rivers Oram Press.

Wellings, K., Field, J., Johnson, A. and Wadsworth, J. (1994) *Sexual Behaviour in Britain: The National Survey of Sexual Attitudes and Lifestyles*. London: Penguin.

Wells, W. (1963) 'How chronic overclaimers distort survey findings.' *Journal of Advertising Research 3*, 8–18.

West London Health Promotion Agency (1994) *Piece By Piece – A Comprehensive Guide to Sexual Health for People with Learning Difficulties*.

Williams, C. (1995) *Invisible Victims: Crime and Abuse against People with Learning Disabilities*. London: Jessica Kingsley Publishers.

Williams, F. (1992) 'Women with learning disabilities are women too.' In M. Langan and L. Day (eds) *Women, Oppression and Social Work*. London: Routledge.

Williams, P. and Shoultz, B. (1982) *We Can Speak for Ourselves*. London: Souvenir Press.

Wistow, G., Knapp, M., Hardy, B. and Allen, C. (1994) *Social Care in a Mixed Economy*. Buckingham: Open University Press.

Wolf, N. (1990) *The Beauty Myth*. London: Vintage.

Wolf, N. (1997) *Promiscuities: A Secret History of Female Desire*. London: Vintage.

Wolfensberger, W. (1972) *The Principle of Normalisation in Human Services*. Toronto: National Institute on Mental Retardation.

Wolfensberger, W. (1983) 'Social role valorization: A proposed new term for the principle of normalisation.' *Mental Retardation 21*, 234–239.

Wyatt, G., Newcomb, M. and Riederle, M. (1993) *Sexual Abuse and Consensual Sex: Women's Developmental Patterns and Outcomes*. Newberry Park, CA: Sage.

Wyngaarden, M. (1981) 'Interviewing mentally retarded persons: Issues and strategies.' In R. Bruininks, C. Meyers, B. Gigford and K. Lakin (eds) *Deinstitutionalisation and Community*

Adjustments of Mentally Retarded People. Monograph 4. Washington, D.C.: American Association on Mental Deficiency.

Young, D. (1996) 'Doing Participatory Action Research with People with Disabilities: Notes from the Field.' Paper presented at the 10th World Congress of International Association for Scientific Study of Intellectual Disability, Helsinki, 8–13 July.

Young People First (1994) *Not Just Painted On: A Report on the First Ever Conference Run by and for People with Down's Syndrome.* London: Young People First.

Subject Index

abortion 47
abuse 24, 69, 175
  see also sexual abuse
acquiescence 97, 98
Adult Training Centres 47
advocacy *see* self-advocacy
Advocacy in Action (support group) 47
Age of Reason and Rationality 42
age of women subjects 121
aggravating circumstances 237, 238
AIDS 65, 66–7, 68, 203
amenorrhea 224
anal sex 139, 141, 205–6, 228, 245
  negative reactions to 142, 148, 205
  taboos on 217, 218
analysis of data 82, 84, 87, 112–13
androcentric bias 88
anonymity 91, 95, 102–4
anthropology 81, 82, 243
arrest of people with learning disability 76
asylums 42, 43, 50
  see also public institutions
attraction 19, 60
Australia 205, 237
autonomy 95
barrier contraception 221, 222
beneficence 95
Beverley Lewis House 77
biological perspectives 18, 58
Black women *see* ethnic minorities
body hair 185, 189, 221
body image 110, 182–7, 220–1, 227
breast screening 223
breasts 142, 185, 206
Britain 45, 46, 47, 54, 60
  studies 71

Canada 210
cap, contraceptive 222, 223

care in the community *see* community care; community settings
celibacy 57, 218
cervical screening 223
child abuse 24, 35, 37, 38, 164, 237
  see also incest
children, parental desire for 125, 161, 196, 219–20
children, sex education for 240, 256
citizen advocacy 47
  see also self-advocacy
civil and human rights *see* human and civil rights
civil law 236, 254
class oppression 34
Cleveland County 37–8
client terminology cycle 44
clitoris 136, 185n, 207, 227, 245
clothes 33, 155, 190–3, 206
coital imperative 23
community care 50, 51, 52
community settings 120, 153, 202, 225–8, 230
  payment for sex in 150, 151, 225
condoms 149, 222, 223, 245
confidants 134–6, 208, 216, 243
  see also friendships; parents; staff
confidentiality 91, 102–4, 232, 239
consent 75, 86, 95, 104–7, 213–14
  research recommendations on 253, 255
CONSENT (sex education team) 65
contact abuse 69
contemporary perspectives 55–67
contraception 56–7, 178, 195–8, 221–5
  Depo-Provera 61, 195, 196, 221, 222, 224
control 49, 127, 226
  of fertility 34, 35, 222
  by staff 134–5, 186, 191, 220
counselling 72, 75, 96, 97

couplehood 216
CPS (Crown Prosecution Service) 235
criminal justice system 76, 236, 246, 247
  justice for women 175
  see also law
critiques 22–30, 39, 85, 251–2
Crown Prosecution Service (CPS) 235

dangerous people, stereotype 53
dark, fear of 150
data analysis 82, 84, 87, 112–13
day services 47, 238
decision making on sexual activity 155–7
deinstitutionalisation 50–2, 230
Denmark 44
Depo-Provera 61, 195, 196, 221, 222, 224
diaphragm, contraceptive 222
discrimination 83, 86
distress 95, 96, 103
domestic violence 60
double disadvantage 86–7
Down's Syndrome 122, 220
dreams 132–4
dress codes, women's 33

eating disorders 189
editing style, data analysis 113
either/or questions 97, 98
elderly people 19
Ellis, Havelock 21, 23, 24
emotion 207, 208
empowerment 49, 99, 244–5, 255
England 50
enjoyment of sexual activity 122–5, 162, 180, 181
equal opportunities 45, 212, 254
erogenous zones 206
erotic education 244
eternal child stereotype 53
ethics 95, 96, 106, 107, 229
ethnic minorities 39, 40, 121, 252–3, 255
  feminists 34
ethnography 80–3, 91
eugenics 54
experiential empowerment 245

Names Index

Thompson, D. (1995) 65, 66, 67, 230, 249

Thompson, D. (1996) 78, 108, 169, 231, 240, 249

Thompson, D. (1997) 16, 38, 69, 71, 72, 73, 76, 78, 106, 107, 210, 212, 215, 232, 233, 234, 246

Thompson, D. (1998) 58, 63, 64, 78, 90, 176, 195, 204, 205, 207, 223, 239, 246, 247, 250

Thompson, S. (1990) 241, 243, 244

Thomson, R. 205, 209, 240

Thomson, X. 244

Tiefer, L. 19, 25, 208

Tonkin, B. 62

Townsend, P. 51

Townsley, R. 84, 106, 253

Trent, J. 15, 16

Troiden, R. 93

Tuke, S. 42

Turk, V. 69, 71, 72, 73, 176, 212, 233, 234

Turner, S. 221

Tymchuk, A. 62

Unger, O. 62

Van Zijderfeld, B. 56

Van Zijerfeld, B. 56

Vance, C. 30

Ventura, J. 142, 207, 209, 216, 228, 241

Ville, I. 83

Walmsley, J. 85, 88, 204, 250

Walsall Women's Group 77

Ward, E. 36

Weber, M. 81

Weeks, J. 19, 20

Wellings, K. et al. 29, 206

Wells, W. 98

West London Health Promotion Agency 67, 137, 205

Whitmore, R. 53

Whittemore, R. 53

Wilkins, R. 69, 71

Wilkinson, D. 126–7, 146

Williams, C. 47, 76, 247

Williams, F. 11, 65, 86, 219, 222, 253

Williams, P. 47

Wise, S. 87, 89, 90, 91

Wistow, G. et al. 14

Wolf, N. 220, 243

Wolfensberger, W. 45, 57, 58

Wyatt, G. 53, 203, 206, 211

Wyngaarden, M. 98, 99, 102, 104

Young, D. 84, 111

Young People First 47